FOR MY MOM AND DAD

FOR HOLDING ME ON THAT FRIDAY NIGHT IN SYNAGOGUE
WHEN THE RABBI SAID:

*"Dear God, please help us to understand why there is
illness and death in our lives. And somewhere in the understanding,
help us to know that there is a blessing in all of this."*

If I grow up I am going to change the world
I am going to be a clown in a circus
I am going to make a wish on every star in the sky

If I grow up I am going to dance on mountaintops
I am going to own two cats
I am going to sing for no reason at all

If I grow up I am going to paint a mural as big as the world
I am going to swim from here to China
I am going to stop to smell the roses

If I grow up I am going to teach people to smile more
I am going to stay up past my bedtime
I am going to write a book

If I grow up I am going to wear clothes that do not match
I am going to sit on the ocean shore and let the waves hit me
I am going to remember every single second
    how wonderful it is to be alive

MEREDITH, AGE 18

Published by:

Scott Fried
P.O. Box 112
Old Chelsea Station
New York, NY 10113

ISBN: 0-9659046-0-1
Printed in the United States of America
Library of Congress Catalog Card Number: 97-90703

Book Design by Laura Herzberg
Back Cover Photo by Andrew Greenspan

For information on how to order more copies of this book or on Scott Fried's lectures, please write to the address above, or call (212) 465-2646

Imagine AIDS as a dark angel

that wrestles with our collective spirit in the existential night.
We struggle to earn our grace as it fractures our
unyielding notions about the invincibility of growing
up. Though we prevail, AIDS refashions our
relationships with life and death and we are

never   ever   the same.

And Jacob was left alone; and a man wrestled with him until the breaking of the day. When the man saw that he did not prevail against Jacob, he touched the hollow of his thigh; and Jacob's thigh was put out of joint as he wrestled with him. Then he said, "Let me go, for the day is breaking." But Jacob said, "I will not let you go, unless you bless me. "

Genesis 32:24-26

The day is breaking,
demand a blessing.

Author's note

When I was a teenager, very few people ever said to me, "It's okay to love yourself exactly as you are. It's okay to love whomever you choose to love. It's okay to believe in yourself and all that you stand for, no matter how different you may feel from everyone else. And it's okay to be confused."

So I have written this book for two specific audiences: teenagers and their parents. First, for teenagers who need to be educated and represented so that no teenager will ever bury his hands in his pockets, look the other way and learn the lessons about life the way I have. And second, for parents and other people who associate with teens, who must be made more aware of the effect of AIDS on today's youth. In addition, this book is for any adult who has forgotten that they too were once a vulnerable teenager themselves.

At different times, interwoven throughout, I am conversing directly with the teens, while at other times I am speaking directly to parents about my conversations with their children. It is my intention that both teenager and parent read each chapter, almost as if one were eavesdropping on the other.

In between the chapters are original poems written by teens themselves. I asked the youngsters to write one of three poems entitled "If I grow up," "If my friend had AIDS," or "This is my prayer as I race under the moon." Included herein are just a few of the hundreds of original poems I have collected over the years.

Some of the names in the following stories have been changed for the sake of confidentiality and anonymity. In certain cases, however, at the teenager's request, I have kept their real name.

The unending process of self-examination and disclosure involved in the writing of this book has been both excruciatingly painful and quite healing, revealing to me in all its rawness, that the wisdom gained and stories gathered from all my searching and lecturing can never take away the threatening consequences of my earlier actions. So I have written this book as both gentle armor and benevolent weapon. In laying down some of the burden of the past few years, I have tried to illustrate my transformation from victim to warrior and turn a curse into a blessing for others to share.

Finally, I have written this book because I needed to read a book like it. Indeed, I am a student of all that I teach.

Many thanks to those friends who helped edit the numerous drafts of this manuscript and who offered advice and support. Thanks mostly to the teens, whose generosity of spirit is unending. I am both graced by and grateful for the earnestness and courage they have so unselfishly shared.

Introduction

This book is a collection of lectures, stories and poems gathered over a period of five years as I traveled around the country to meet with tens of thousands of teenagers. They are lectures to, stories of and poems by teenagers learning about HIV/AIDS in high schools, colleges and universities, churches and synagogues, youth groups, conferences, retreats and on the streets - anywhere and everywhere young people congregate. For purposes of telling their stories, the setting for this book takes place at a series of summer camps over the period of a single summer.

My intention has been to talk to the teens about how I got infected with HIV and to share my message of hope and courage with as many of them as possible. My aim was to convey, in short, that in order to learn how to stay safe, one must first learn *why* to stay safe.

As I started sharing this body of work with my adult friends, one of them, Shaun, shared with me his insight:

> *When teaching teenagers about AIDS, you must draw upon an incredible capacity to*
> *love while staying completely in the moment; be present. You must be able to pay attention.*
> *Notice and note the small intricacies all the rest of us glance over quickly, hurrying on*
> *our way. You must mark each moment. When you are with teenagers, pay attention.*
> *Pay homage to their emotions and their concerns and their whole process of explanation.*
> *Take time to give time...to return time robbed or taken away by others less willing.*
> *Be willing, my friend, and you will succeed.*

Teenagers ask many questions. In my travels, I discovered what they are really asking behind their careful wording. "Is it safe to be alive?" "Can I hold onto hope?" "Will you look me in the eyes and tell me the truth?" They ask the world of me, giving me their hope in return for a chance to be free from their fear. It has been my privilege to do more than simply offer them answers; I try to return their hope with compassion, and by doing so, together somehow we'll find our way.

These teens present the clearest vision of the memory of promises I made at their age — promises to always remain pure of purpose with the unblemished expectation that love is what's needed in order to grow up. In the meantime, a silent promise is made: "this moment is enough and the memory of this moment I shall carry with me always."

When I teach teenagers about AIDS it is easy for me to believe in some greater good of which I am a part. If I am still and attentive I can feel the movement of energy between us. Love. The kind of love I believed in at their age. They either carry it with them or they awaken it in me. Perhaps both. And at once I know that my presence in their lives is a lasting one. I am immortalized in their collective memory, and it heals me.

If it could be said that all eternity exists in a single pure moment, then together these teens and I have shared something that will last beyond time itself. More than simply my students, they have become my teachers, mentors and friends. Through them, I have learned about the privilege of assisting in a child's development. Moreover, they remind me to see the world more clearly with the same wide-eyed passion for living that youth embraces.

As my friend Deborah describes it, "The true work is to uncover people's magnificence so that they can know it in themselves and see it in others." It is my hope, thereby, that my brief presence in their lives will help them to recognize, cherish and value their own. For this is indeed what they have taught me.

At the end of my travels, I met a woman who asked me, in Hebrew, "Ma Yesh?" I think she meant it as a greeting, but in my broken understanding of the language, I took it to mean, "What do you have?"

"Stories," I said. "Lots and lots of stories."

These are some of them. ❧

I

my story

Gentle Scott, your story is our story   *Do you see?*
That is our connection - our reflection
In your mortal struggle for love and holiness
Be strong in spirit   —Shirah, age 24

On Monday night, November 30, 1987, with the memory of Thanksgiving weekend, family and food still fresh in my mind, I took the #1 subway uptown to the 72nd Street station. As I exited the train and stepped onto the subway platform, I noticed a newsstand that was gated up and closed for the night. Yet I could still see the front page of the day's unsold New York Daily News and New York Post behind the gates. As I dug my hands deep into the pockets of my favorite ripped jeans, my eyes were drawn to the letters written in boldface and black ink, staring straight back at me:

AIDS

I looked the other way.

With my face bowed to the ground, I took a deep breath, told myself this would be the only time I would ever do this and headed for the fifth floor walk-up on Columbus Avenue and 70th Street where a man I had met only a few weeks before and barely knew would meet me in the vestibule of his building. With a crooked smile and squeeze of my buttocks, he would lead me up the narrow and winding stairwell to the little room on the top floor, with the makeshift loft bed and bare bulb hanging from the ceiling. He would then persuade me to have unsafe sex.

For the following six weeks I performed the same ritual. Once a week, six more times, I took the #1 train uptown, hands in pockets, neck bent and face concealed on the long walk to his apartment, always telling myself that this would be the last time I would ever do this.

"Just this once," I'd say to myself. "I promise the next time I'll be safer and learn to say "no" - convincingly. And he'll believe me. And he'll respect me. And I'll have grown. I promise. Next time. Next time."

And always, as I passed that newsstand, gated up and closed for the night, I looked the other way.

I hated the long forsaken walks toward Columbus and 70th. I hated the broken banister at the top of the stairs. I hated the brown couch against the wall by the window and the music he played and the jeans he always wore, strategically ripped at the crotch. I hated his crooked smile and his pockmarked face and his half-grown beard. Mostly, though, I hated how unsafe I felt every time he called me "Partner."

But this was the first time I was ever "with" another man. The first time any man had ever broken the sacred boundary of personal space I successfully encased around me; my sanctuary from society's guilty verdict handed down to me for experiencing disparate feelings that seemed aberrant, unnatural and wrong. It was the first time anyone had ever said, "I know your secret. It's safe with me."

And it thrilled me.

I loved the ominous way he smelled, and the shifty way he stood too close to me and the dangerous feeling of his bare flesh against mine.

And I hated myself for loving these things. So I turned my head and looked the other way.

"I think we should talk...about...you know...AIDS," I said.

"Okay," he said.

"Do you...know about it?"

"Yeah," he assured me. "I have many friends who've died."

I sat down on the brown couch as he reached for a photo album. He sat down next to me and opened it to a page with pictures of bearded men with beer bellies posing in front of their motorcycles. And as pointed to the ones who had died, I thought to myself, "This is good. He knows about AIDS so I don't have to find out for myself. I can trust his knowledge. I can trust him."

"So have you been...tested?" I asked as I looked away from the book.

"Many times," he said. "Every six months, in fact."

I studied the strange circles under his eyes and the blotches in his skin and the scars on his face and wondered how they all got there. Then, timidly I asked, "Why every six months?"

He explained that he was born with syphilis and often needed to get a check-up, and while at the clinic the doctors would give him an HIV antibody test. I believed him. Because I wanted to believe him.

As I looked out the window into the dark and cold of that late November night I thought to myself, "That's it! I had the conversation about AIDS and I survived it," never once turning back to look him fully in the face and ask if his test results for HIV were negative or positive.

Once a week I took the #1 subway uptown to the apartment at the top of the stairs. To the stifled conversations. To the lure of our aloneness. To the self-imposed shame of sexual capitulation. Once a week, surrendering to his menacing advances, I would try to deny my feelings of being in danger and search for clues that he really did care for me. And that maybe one day, he could even love me. And once a week, lying next to his body, as he reached his arm over my head, I would listen for the sound of plastic, for the unwrapping of a condom from its packet. Sometimes I would hear it; sometimes I wouldn't. But each time with a strange mixture of longing and fear I would say to myself, "This is the last time," and turn my head and look the other way.

⬤

It would be eight more years before I could answer a teenager named Staci sitting in the front row of one of my lectures, who in the middle of hearing me tell my story, with tears streaming down her face and acceptance in her voice, screamed out, "Why, Scott, why?"

2

It took that many years for me to learn to say, "Because I didn't know you then. Because I didn't know my story would hurt you so. And because I didn't know I was worthy of being so loved by someone I barely know."

And it would be years after my unsafe encounter that I would run into "my partner's" neighbor on a street in the West Village. We talked about those weeks back in the winter of 1987.

"I used to come over when I heard you next door," Jordan said. "I wanted to tell you to leave. I wanted to put a sign over his head that read, "AIDS! GET OUT!" But I couldn't get your attention. You were always looking down."

"I didn't want any witnesses that I was ever there," I answered. "I didn't want to even admit it to myself." And then I asked him, "Do you think it would have made any difference?"

"Probably not," he answered. "You were like a moth in a flame. You seemed to have some sort of death wish back then."

"Not a death wish," I responded. "But certainly a lack of a life wish."

I looked straight into Jordan's eyes for the first time, paused for a second and then spoke.

"Did he infect you too?"

"I'm pretty sure it was him," he answered.

My alluring stranger-turned-partner on 70th and Columbus died of AIDS two years ago. Jordan died of AIDS two months ago.

I am still here.

When I was a teenager, I had an eighteen year-old friend who was a soldier in the Israeli army. Hila used to share with me some of her feelings about the possibility of fighting in a war, and about the possibility of fighting for her life. "You must always remember from whence you came," she would say.

"Why, Hila, why?" I would ask.

"Because...you can never defend your future if you can't honor your past."

There are no more witnesses to the events of the winter of 1987. No one left to unravel my lies and reveal my secrets. No one to betray my confidences or tell my story. No one...except me.

And so I share my story as a way of honoring and bearing witness to my past. I share my story in order to stare HIV in the face and find the courage to defend and embrace my future. And finally, I share my story so that when I take the #1 subway uptown and pass that newsstand, gated up and closed for the night, I no longer look the other way. ❧

ALEX

"Look! There's your red moon!" Alex cried when he saw me coming down the hill.

"Race ya to the top," I shouted. "We can see it better from there."

So we positioned our sneakers toe to toe, marked our target in the distance and tore off to get a perfect view of the blood-red full moon of July as it rose in the sky.

Catching our breath, we stood for a few moments at the top of the slope. Wide-eyed and winded, we looked to the sky and silently shared the falling of night.

"I always pray under a full moon," I said, breaking the silence.

"Really?" he asked. "What do you pray for?"

"I secretly say, 'Thanks God. I get it.'"

Alex turned his face away from the sky to look at me.

"That moon is shining just for me," I explained. "God put it there just for me. It's His way of reminding me to keep on believing in life."

It was early evening at summer camp. I was originally there to talk to the campers about AIDS. But on this night, I was being initiated into their club, called the "The Shoafim," which translated from Hebrew means, "Those who aspire."

The first task was the trust walk. Ambling our way around the grounds, we were blindfolded and chained to each other: hand to shoulder, heart to heart. Touching, laughing, setting aside all inhibitions and simply making noise in the night air, we proclaimed our aliveness.

"I claim the moon!" I screamed inside. "I am still alive!"

The next task was to recite out loud, "I am a link in the Shoafim chain, and I promise to ....."

"...to remember you always," I declared.

Many years ago, I sat under the same summer sky, newly diagnosed with HIV. I was alone and afraid, wanting to share all that was happening to me and all I was becoming; wanting to share the blood-red moon of July.

And now I have. For on this night, after freeing a firefly caught in a blade of grass, I rolled down a hill with a group of animated teenagers. Surrendering my favorite pair of ripped jeans to grass stains and dirt, I shouted wishes at the sky.

I raced under the moon.

On this night, I added to my inner refuge of gentle remembrances the Shoafim girls in their bunk, painting their nails and braiding each other's hair. It was after bedtime as I sang them a lullaby, my favorite Jimmy Webb song:

> *When the last moon is cast over the last star of morning*
> *When the future has passed without even a last desperate warning*
> *Then look into the sky where through the clouds a path is born*
> *Look and see her, how she sparkles, it's the last unicorn*
> *I'm alive*

"I'm happy that you are having a good time," whispered one sleepy girl.

"Yeah," added another. "Now you will have fun memories of your visit here."

Still another said, "I think you are a beautiful person. I see that in myself now. No one is better than me. No one can hurt me. You taught me how to recognize myself. You taught me how to love."

If I grow up
I will always watch the full moon of July

I will make a new friend every day
I will write letters to old friends
I will visit every state

The sky and the stars and the moon will be appreciated
  by everyone

I will try to share my feelings
I will tell my brother I love him
I will make a collage of the faces of love

If I grow up
I will never forget a moment

I will play cheezy '80s songs at top volume
I will get people to love nature
Red will stay my favorite color
I will touch the lives of many people

If I grow up
I will always love the sky,
But not so much as I love the full moon of July

KATIE, AGE 16

2

love

On his deathbed, my friend Larry looked around at all the faces looking back
at him, and all the hands being laid on his body, and said, "I'm in so much pain -
more pain than I've ever felt in my whole life. And yet I also feel so much love.
So much pain and so much beauty - all in one day."

—Larry 1956 -1991

What's the first word that comes to mind when you hear the word AIDS? Just call it out.

DEATH   PAIN   LOSS   SORROW   DEPRESSION   TRAGEDY   SICKNESS   FEAR

That's right. We've all heard a lot about those words, which are certainly a part of AIDS. But there's another side to AIDS as well. A side rarely spoken about. When I hear the word AIDS, the first word I think of is...LOVE.

Ironically, one of the blessings HIV/AIDS has brought me is the abundance of love right here in this room. Certainly, the need for it exists. AIDS has inspired me to get a bunch of really terrific teenagers together to sit around and talk about our feelings. We are doing what needs to be done. And in so doing, we are creating a certain kind of cure.

There is a healing around AIDS that exists when we look into each other's eyes and when we really communicate with each other. We can learn to say, "I'm not afraid to be near you if you are HIV+. I'm not afraid of you because you are like me. You have the same dreams as I do." AIDS prompts us to say, "Hey, I care about you and I want to make sure that you stay alive. I'll do what I can."

In every generation there has been something that characterizes the inner struggle of the general masses. AIDS is ours. And as with every struggle, there is always an emancipation, something that needs to be liberated or loosened from our collective spirit. In coming together and learning how to care for each other we are liberating the love within us, the love that heals.

In its purest form, we all experience love on some level, in every day of our lives, though we may not always realize it. In fact, it's why we've come together today. So when we talk about AIDS, we need to also talk about love. This doesn't necessarily take AIDS away, but it does make room for it in our world. Room for the acceptance of the need to be educated. Room for the deep level of compassion and understanding needed in order to remember our oneness. Room for each other. Like what we're doing here in this room today - educating people, enlightening people, encouraging people to function from more of an emotional place.

When we turn our faces away from AIDS, we are also turning our faces away from each other. And all we've got is each other. Whatever it is we do, we are sharing this life together.

AIDS is a part of that sharing. AIDS draws us closer and helps us to understand each other more. The words you all mentioned before, like death, pain and sorrow, were brought up because you understand something about them from your own life experiences. Indeed, everyone in this room has experienced some sort of pain or life challenge, whatever it is. We all want to help each other. It's no different if you are HIV positive or HIV negative.

AIDS makes people talk.

Indeed, everyone is thinking about it, and everyone has something to say about it. Most of us even have the same questions. What's more important to me than even giving you the answers is giving you the opportunity to find out that you have questions. Then at least you'll know that you have the right to ask. It's not so much in knowing the answers that we learn. It's in opening up enough to talk that we learn, because we feel safer when we talk. Words have the power to help us feel safe.

AIDS gets us in touch with the moment at hand, so that we live in the moment and hope the moments will last for a long, long time. I still want the things that you want for yourselves: a life well-lived with all my dreams coming true. One of those dreams is to see an army of teenagers across this country and around this world, that are changing the general perception of AIDS from ignorance to education, from fear to motivation, and from loss to love. 🦎

> **I think that love is a cure.**
> **If someone loves you,**
> **you feel better.**
>
> —*Chris, Age 11*

BUNK 6

It is midnight. Past curfew. Past lights out. I am participating in a "sharing circle" with seven girls seated on the floor of their cabin. We are imparting our innermost secrets, disclosing insecurities for the very first time to each other. Picking candle wax drippings off the wooden slates of the floor, we whisper to one another as the shadows from the dim light of the candle amply hide our faces, making us feel safe enough to confess and reveal.

Randy is fourteen. She is overweight and unhappy. "I feel that nobody can understand my mood swings. I just want you all to know that I am trying."

"Has anyone ever told you that you are fine the way you are, Randy?" I hear myself ask. She shrugs one shoulder as she plays with the melting wax on the candle.

"Why don't we all whisper it to her so she can keep it in her memory when she needs it?" And a hushed chorus of thirteen year-old sopranos softly proclaim: "You are fine the way you are, Randy."

Janie, who doesn't like her voice because she thinks it is too deep, is afraid to speak her opinions. Julie thinks others are talking about her behind her back. Lisa never really learned how to open up to anyone. Melissa is shy. Sherry thinks she is fat. And Erica is embarrassed to wear a bathing suit for fear of revealing a "huge scar from a kidney operation."

Seven girls, who hardly knew one another's last names at the start of day, are now eager to offer up their weaknesses for all to embrace. And I, as witness to this fresh courage, begin to believe that the rare disclosure and acceptance of what we think of as inner flaws soon become the inner anchors and even magnets of our personalities as we grow. The more weaknesses — if they be so called — that we embrace within, perhaps the more incorruptible we can become.

Randy scribbles something on a piece of paper, and hands it to me as I leave their cabin. On it she has written the words,

> *"Bright and gold of sunlight and silver,*
> *You taught me there is always a rose in a fisted glove."*

9

In a world of fear and carelessness
Where best friends can turn into bitter enemies
When the hurt and heartbroken have nowhere to turn
It is my wish for the forlorn and the lost
The scared and the wicked
And all those who have lost
And will lose
To have a place to turn to
Someone who will care and nourish
And raise hope from despair

ANONYMOUS

3

"no"

*"AIDS is not what's gonna kill you, even if your test results come back positive.
What'll kill you is that you don't know how to say 'no'. That's what's gonna kill you!"*

—My HIV test counselor

OK. You are all between eleven and twelve years of age, is that right?
Do you all know why I'm here today?

Maybe because when you were a kid, you went to this camp?

That's a good guess. But no, I went to day camp as a kid. So who else has an idea
about why I'm here?

You're going to talk to us about AIDS.

That's exactly right! But before we talk about AIDS, I want to ask you a few questions about
yourselves. Who can tell me what it means to have self-confidence and self-esteem?

To trust your instincts.

To not be influenced by other people.

To be proud of yourself and keep your head high.

Don't be afraid to say "no."

Good. Having self-confidence and self-esteem means not being afraid to say "no".
But before you can learn how to say "no" you have to first know why to say "no". Right?
So who can tell me why to say "no"?

Because you could get hurt if you don't.

Good. Someone else. Why do you say "no"?

Because you wanna keep yourself healthy and happy.

Because it's the right thing to do.

Why is it the right thing to do?

Because it's what you believe.

And why is it what you believe?

Because it feels good inside.

And why does it feel good inside when you do what you believe, like saying "no"? I'll tell you. Because you're worth it.

That's why you say "no". Because you're worth it!

Who can give me an example of when you'd want to say "no"?

When somebody offers you drugs.

Someone offers you drugs and you want to say "no." Good. How do you do it? Listen carefully to each other; your friends are going to teach you something today.

You should say "no", but also teach them that it also isn't very good for them.

So you're saying "no" in a nice way, as an educator. All right. Good for you. What's another way of saying "no"?

Um, a broken record.

For those of us who don't know what you mean, could you explain that?

Saying "no" over and over again.

You could try saying, "Let me think about it first."

Alright! And then really think about it. No, do more than that. Talk about it. Think out loud in front of a friend.

A great way is, you could ask somebody else to help you to say "no."

More. I want more. How do you say "no"?

Say, "It's not for me."

You could say, "It's time for dinner, gotta go!" or "I have other plans."

You could say to the other person, "Get a life!"

Or you could just walk away.

Good. It's all good. How about another time when you would want to say "no"?

Like...if you have a really good friend and they want to have sex with you and you don't want to have sex with them.

I see...when somebody asks you to do something you don't feel comfortable doing, like drugs or unsafe sex or any kind of sex at all.

But what if your friends force you do something?

Okay, now here's a good question. Tell me something a friend would force you do. What's on your mind?

Like if they threaten me to do drugs.

Okay. Anybody here have an answer for that one?

Well, if they want you do something that you don't want to do, then they're not really your friends.

That's a good answer. Listen up. When I was a teenager, saying "no" wasn't an option. Each time I tried to say it, it never made a difference. So in addition to learning how to say "no", learn to *hear* "no". Respect other peoples' wishes. Remember, we're talking about AIDS and you. I'm not talking about criminals. I'm not talking about strangers. I'm not talking about dangerous people. I'm talking about your friends. How do you say "no?"

[Everybody screams] No!!!
Let me hear it again! No!!!
One more time! No!!!

Okay. That's great! But for some of us, just saying "no" is still difficult. So what do you do then? I'm going to teach you another way to "Just Say No." But I want to know that you all hear me. So everybody, scream with me: "YES."

YES!!!

Excellent.

One way to "just say no" to someone else is by learning how to say "yes" to yourself.

"No" to somebody else starts with "yes" to yourself. If you don't want to have sex with somebody, or if you don't want to have unprotected sex with somebody, or if you don't want to do drugs, or if you don't want to smoke, or if you don't want to get in a car with somebody who is drunk, or if you don't want to hang out with a group of people that you don't feel good about, or if you don't want to do something because your inner voice knows better, or *whatever*, saying "no" to those people starts with saying "yes" to yourself. Because when you say "yes" to yourself, it makes it easier to say "no" to somebody else.

"Yes, I care about myself."

"Yes, I care about my life."

"Yes, I am feeling uncomfortable."

"Yes, I need more time to decide."

"Yes, I can say 'no.'"

But first you have to know who it is you are saying "yes" to. You have to know how to like yourself and care about yourself. Does anyone here really like themselves? You do? How do you know?

13

I won't do other things that I'm not ready for.
I think that I'm pretty.
I'm proud of the things that I do and the things that I accomplish.

What are some other things you're proud of?

Doing good in school.
Being accepted for who I am.
I'm proud of having friends.

And what does having friends mean to you?

I know that people like me. There must be something good about me if people like me.

I like that. I like that a lot.

I respect myself.

How do you respect yourself?

By treating myself well.

And how do you treat yourself well?

By making the right choices.

And how do you make the right choices?

By believing in myself.

That's good. It's all good. Everybody put your hands down for a minute and look at me. Shhh! Listen carefully. Can you all see me? Okay. Can you all see that I have brown hair? I'm wearing a white T-shirt and ripped jeans. I'm 5'3" and I have three string bracelets on my left wrist. You all see that, right? Well, what you can't see is that I'm also HIV+.

I came here this morning to tell you that treating yourselves well, making the right choices and believing in yourselves are some of the most important things you can ever learn. If you learn, as you say in your own words, to "hold your head up high, believe in yourselves and not be afraid to say 'no,'" then chances are you won't become infected with HIV. These are some of the most important things you can learn in order to keep yourself alive.

As you grow older, learn as much as you can about AIDS. You know a lot now. In fact, you know a lot more about AIDS than some adults I know. Don't stop learning. Teach yourselves. Teach each other. Don't be scared; be brave. Learn. Read. Ask. Talk. Listen. OK?

Before you got infected, did you believe in yourself?

No, I think that's one of the reasons I got infected. Do *you* believe in yourself?

Yes. 🐝

14

KATIE

"It's people like you," Katie said during lunch, "that make the sky seem blue and the sun shine bright. I just want to tell you that you inspired me to live my life to the fullest and love every minute of it."

Katie is fifteen and reminds me of the image I created in my mind of the character Scout, after reading *To Kill a Mockingbird* for the first time. Some would call her a tomboy, but I see her as a gorgeous little girl with a unique vitality and a charmed sense of who she is and who she will be when she grows up.

Katie thinks she can find a cure for AIDS by simply taking out the bad blood and exchanging it for good blood. "I mean, think about it," she says. "It makes sense. Really. I don't see why it can't be done."

She just might do it one day.

Katie is also a singer, with a young alto voice and quick vibrato that instantly settles the mind and grabs at the heart. She wrote me a song today and sang it to me as I was reaching across her arm for a napkin during lunch. Unrestrained and proud, her voice rang out over the cacophony of the feasting hungry campers:

> *You know I love you, every minute of the day*
> *You know I love you, you make the storm clouds go away*
> *The world is always turning*
> *And the stars are always burning*
> *And my heart is always beating*
> *Love*

Katie is always singing.

If I grow up
I want to find a hidden waterfall
Or see a sunset where nobody has ever seen it from before

I'd like to sit on top of a mountain that nobody has been to the top of
And see the view for myself
I'd like to pet a lion
And when I was done
I'd know that I was the only one who would ever pet that lion

I want to find that one most incredible sight
That will never be found by anyone else
And admire it in complete awe
Because when the day comes when everyone will see
What I am not able to see
I'll always remember that I've seen sights
And have been to places
That they will never have the privilege of seeing

REBECCA, AGE 16 – diagnosed with retinitis pigmentosa
(retinal degeneration that can cause blindness)

4

denial

"While I was in the clinic, waiting for some tests, I saw a guy with KS lesions on his face. And instead of following my impulse to turn away, I stuck out my hand and said, "My name's Carl. What's yours?" I mean, if I can't embrace AIDS, then I can't help myself to recover."

—A share at one of my HIV support groups

Imagine you're a normal middle-class kid, just out of college, excited about life and looking for a job. You get the flu, or something like it. You go to the doctor and he recommends that you have an HIV antibody test; the test results come back positive. Can't happen to you? Somebody wrote on this blackboard behind me, with exclamation marks: "It will never happen to me!" I've got news for you - I thought the same thing, too, until it did. How many of you in this room know people who are putting themselves at risk for HIV infection?

Keep your hands up and take a look around. There is not one person in this room of four hundred teenagers that doesn't have a hand up. This is a frightening sight.

I'm not here to scare you. But I am here to scare you. So tell me the truth. Why are you not protecting yourselves?

"It will never happen to me!"

Teenagers think they're invincible and that nothing can happen to them.

When you say it can't happen to you, 99 percent is a feeling of invincibility and 1 percent is not caring enough about yourself to pay attention to that little voice in the back of your brain that says, "Yes it can!"

A lot of times you end up doing things because things happen and you don't even think twice.

You mean, one thing leads to another and before you know it you're in trouble. Like, you're having too many drinks and you're not able to articulate your needs or even get away. Or you don't have enough self-confidence to say what it is that you want or don't want. Or maybe you're just having a good time and you think, "Hey, I don't care. I'll throw caution to the wind. I'll think about it in six months when I get my test results back."

I guess I'm scared of having to deal with it. I'm scared of exactly what you said, like, not being able to say something. I've always been a strong person with my feelings, but actions are a different story.

Back when I got infected, I thought one way about myself and then went ahead and behaved in a totally different way. Can any of you relate to that? Many of us have a secret life. We convince ourselves that we feel a certain way when we really don't. And sometimes we know better and still we close our eyes. As one teenager says, "We ride rough shots with our feelings."

I think when you're young, you really think you're immortal. You just don't think that anything will happen to you. I mean, when you're 17 or whatever, you just don't think about death, you know.

Basically, I was just like everyone else. I never really thought it could happen to me. I always heard about AIDS but I didn't know much about it. Then I went to see the movie "Philadelphia" with some of my friends. I really figured this isn't real, only ignorant hicks think that only gays get it and they deserved to get it. I didn't think that any of my friends could feel that way with all the education that we have. But when I left the movie, my date was saying that the guy in the movie did deserve it. What ignorance!

People that I know and people just like me feel that AIDS is a disease that they can't get and AIDS is something that is shameful.

I really want to help people understand, to tell them that the ignorance has to stop. And as soon as ignorance stops, then the AIDS virus hopefully will disappear.

Wow! And what is ignorance, really?

A lack of knowledge.

Right. And what comes with a lack of knowledge?

A fear of the unknown.

So maybe people think, "It can't happen to me," because of ignorance or fear of the unknown.

Maybe they know that it can happen to them and they don't want to face it, like saying, "Go away" and maybe it will.

Right. Whether we think that we're different or separate or immune - we're not. We all have to deal with this. And we all have to deal with ourselves.

A lot of times, um, people hate in others what they hate in themselves.

Before I got infected, part of me hated myself, too. I remember writing in my diary one night, "As surely as God must laugh at my jokes, He must be crying from how much I dislike myself?" I thought it was bad to be confused. I thought I was the only one who felt that way. Looking back, I can see there was nothing wrong with those thoughts. What was wrong was thinking something was wrong with them. I was unsure and ashamed of my sexuality. Heterosexuality. Homosexuality. Bisexuality. Whatever! I was scared of the whole notion of sexuality. And I was not sure where love fit in. Even though I was beginning to come to terms with my feelings, I sought out an encounter that confirmed the majority of my shame and low self-esteem. I found somebody that was kind of dangerous so I'd affirm for myself that it's the wrong thing to do. I put myself in a situation where I could act out my denial and self-hate. And while I was having unsafe sex, I remember thinking to myself, "These are the arms I deserve around me." I truly didn't want to feel good about it. I felt that I had to pay a price just for being alive. Can anyone here relate?

Like I look at the veins in your arm and then I look at the veins in my arm, and, like, they're the same veins, but the blood that's running through them... I mean... we're so much the same, and well...

If there's anything that sticks in my mind it is that HIV doesn't discriminate.

It doesn't discriminate against race. It doesn't discriminate against religion. And it doesn't discriminate against sex. It's a "people disease." People, as in the whole world.

Anybody in the world.

You know, I took health class just to get the easy grade. I didn't really care what the teacher said. I never listened. I don't even remember his name. But this definitely puts everything into perspective and I know now that I have to be safe. It's my life and I'd like it to be a long one.

It's so frustrating to see that there are people out there who know about AIDS and they know how you get it but they're not doing anything to prevent it.

It's important to try to figure out why they're not doing anything with this knowledge. Why is it that some people live in denial? What are they wrestling with? Where does their fear come from that it cripples them so?

It's not as if we don't have enough problems already in the world, you know? It's just one more major problem. I mean, we're going into the 21st century with problems with the environment and over-population, plus this now. So many problems. As a kid, you don't really think about it. But then you grow up and hear about it and you know you're gonna have to deal with it.

You survive because you have to. You learn the skills because you have to. I think that too many people are afraid to talk this openly. Yet the more you learn to speak up, the more you know what your questions are. If you can at least take with you into the world the questions you've got, somewhere there'll be an answer.

But some people still don't talk about it. Like, when this other girl came back from college, she said that so many people were having unprotected sex and it was just no big deal. Not only am I concerned for myself, but there's so many other people that don't know. They just have no clue. Are there people that I'm gonna encounter that have no clue about this?

Yes. And so your job is a little tougher because you are learning about the facts. And once you know them, it's hard to keep your mouth shut. I'm not saying be a crusader, but — be a crusader. Knowledge of this stuff brings with it responsibility to others.

I am sick and tired of turning on the news every day and looking in the paper and seeing AIDS written all over the place. I can't understand it, you know, since we can control whether or not we can contract the virus. It's not something like the common cold. If you put yourself at risk, you get it. If you don't put yourself at risk, then you don't get it. And yet it's still wiping out populations and... it's just horrible.

I guess I'm scared of having to deal with it myself. I think that all of us in this room can say that because, you know, we're high risk. Just, like, being told that we're high risk is scary.

Try to have compassion for yourselves. When you feel an unfamiliar darkness, remember the faces in this room today. Know that we're afraid for a reason. Let's work on this together. Together we can turn the fear into education and motivation. Right? Are you all with me? As we educate ourselves and each other we find out what is safe and what is not safe. Then the fear doesn't stop us or halt our growth anymore. In fact, then it actually promotes our growth.

What is the point of fear if it doesn't help us to grow?

So the way out is to educate, to communicate and to care. To care about each other. To care about the people in this room. To care about the people you have sex with. To care enough to say, "I'll look after you if you'll look after me. I'll remember you if you'll remember me." Yeah, it's embarrassing, yeah, it's corny, yet it just might save your lives.

I may never see any of you again, yet you are teaching me something I can teach so many other people.

It's up to our generation. It is our responsibility to put an end to it, or try to at least, you know.

Together, we are becoming people who save lives, including our own. ❧

ETAI

Etai is seventeen and has Cerebral Palsy.

His large wheelchair was egregiously placed in front of me during my Saturday night lecture. As I talked about my trials and thanksgiving, he was moved to testify about some of his own.

"It's not easy. And you get frustrated and down," he started to say to the room. "But the point is, these experiences are what make us who we are. I think the Cerebral Palsy makes me who I am, and I love it. I love the chair. I do. I really do."

"Because you love yourself," I submitted.

"Because I love myself and because I see that I have such a unique view of the world and I don't think anybody else but me has this exact view."

"The curiosity is," he continued, "I wonder if you, being HIV positive, see it the same way. And I see that you do. I mean, I can feel it from you that you see so much more than anybody else here. The words are escaping me now, but I think it's great. Do you follow what I'm saying?"

"I think we all do," I answered.

And in that moment, I remembered one of my teachers once saying to me, "If you see it in others, it must first be somewhere in yourself." So with those words, I spoke to the room.

"For any of you right now who are moved by what Etai has just said, it means to me that you too have the same specialness. It takes one to know one. Every single one of us is capable of experiencing what Etai is talking about — a passion for life with a reverence for the immediacy of the moment, a recognition of the beauty in the frailty of our bodies, and an understanding that everything we need is given to us in each moment if we believe and have faith enough to open our hearts. Yes, Etai?"

"Yes. Most definitely. Most definitely."

After my talk, he wheeled himself over to me to extend his blessings. "I believe that you will have all the desires of your heart," he offered, "because you have so much to give."

"And you, Etai? What about your heart?"

"I have just two wishes," he answered. "Even though I am comfortable with the CP, I wish that people could see me sitting in the chair, instead of just the chair. And I wish that I could have a date on a Saturday night."

"You know something, Etai?" I offered. "I've always felt that we praise God every time our hearts break."

"Why?" he asked, looking up at me from his chair.

"Because it shows that we are using to the fullest potential the heart which He has so carefully entrusted unto us."

"I see," he answered. "Yes, I see."

"And you know something else, Etai?" I continued. "I believe that you too one day will have all the desires of your heart, because you have so much to give."

Love is dripping away from the earth
  showing up in the strangest places

Love is a rare animal
  hiding from hurtful people

And love, at the same time
  is touching the heart of innocent people

  I am hoping for love
  leaning on love
  reaching out to love
  encouraging it
  saving it
  treasuring it
  running after it,
  running after it

JENI, AGE 15

5

abstinence

Dear Scott, hi. I'm not sure if you remember me. But I felt the need to write to you. You spoke tonight at my camp and I walked you to the parking lot. There is a lot I wanted to say to you but I am very shy, and I felt I could do it better on paper. If it all doesn't make sense, I'm sorry.

Let me tell you a little bit about myself. I am eighteen years old and very naive. I've had very little experience sexually. I feel very alone and very unsure of who I am. Everything that I've always enjoyed doing no longer interests me. I basically have no idea of who I am. Like I said before, I am very shy, but you made me feel like I wasn't the only person in the world who felt like this. I felt compelled to tell you. I wish you only the best. Truly, Alisa

—A camper in the northeast

Abstinence, abstinence, abstinence is good, good, good, for three reasons;

    1) because I was told to teach you that;

    2) because it's the safest form of sex, and

    3) because you don't have to have sex if you don't want to have sex.

Whatever the reason;

        if you are not ready

        if it goes against your cultural beliefs

        if it goes against your religious beliefs

        if you are waiting until you get married

        if it doesn't feel right

        if something else seems more important

        if you are afraid

        if you are simply not interested

        if proper protection isn't available

        if you don't want a one-night stand

        if you haven't met the right person

        if your partner hasn't been tested

        if you want to know more about your partner

        if you want your partner to know more about you

if you want to explore other aspects of the relationship

if you're afraid that it might ruin the relationship

if you promised your parents you'd wait

if your hormones haven't kicked in yet

if you are too busy studying for your SAT's

if you would rather try out for the track team

if you had a negative sexual experience in the past

if you have already had sex and would like to return to waiting

or any other reason you might have

then you don't have to have sex.

When I was in high school, it seemed like a lot of my friends were having sex. But I never really knew whether or not they were telling the truth. I knew that I wasn't ready to have sex but there was nobody around to say, "Hey, that's cool," in spite of the peer pressure. If you fall into this category,

I'm here to represent your feelings. It's okay.

You are not uncool or a square or a faggot or a loser or a reject or bad or behind schedule or missing out or immature or anything if you aren't having sex.

Just because we're talking about sex doesn't mean you have to have sex.

THE BLIND MAN

Last night I met a blind man. He was sitting in the corner of the room at my Tuesday HIV/AIDS support group, sharing with us the difficulty he was having navigating his body on the streets of the city. He explained how he waited for people to offer assistance, knowing that they probably wouldn't, and told us how much difference a simple "Can I help?" would have made.

"Some blind people," he said, "don't want to be assisted." I suppose he meant that they are comfortable and confident. "But my blindness is AIDS related and it's all so new to me, and I need help."

And I began to think about the night I hailed a cab for a blind lady. It was Christmas Eve and though the night was full, the streets were vacant. I wanted to tell her that, while her arm was superfluously extended, a cab was idling in front of her.

But I was afraid.

And as I sat through last night's meeting, I thought about our fear of people who are different and why we don't offer assistance often enough. Until a blonde-haired man with cancer sitting on a couch to my right, shared his take on it. He said he too is afraid to help blind people, but that his fear is not of that which is unfamiliar or appearing inferior or a reminder of the breakable within us all.

"What if I don't do it right?" he asked. "What if, as I walk you across the street, I put you in some kind of danger?"

And at once I recognized the insecurity of goodness. For maybe sometimes what seems like discrimination is only a matter of perception. Maybe fear-based actions are not always the result of negative thinking. Sometimes, they can be the response of a soft and timid heart.

The blind man in the corner thanked the blonde man on the couch and the room applauded. And I began to think that perhaps it is in the acceptance of our imperfections that maybe we are as perfect as we'll ever be.

A star full of skies
Over an open field
Where I can chase dandelions

A cedar house
With a high-beamed roof
On a faded mountain back

In my love's arms
Through summer blooms we walk

On the porch
In a wicker rocker
Of falling autumn leaves we watch

JESSLYN, AGE 15

6

safer sex

A part of sexual activity is feelings. I'd say the biggest part. Even 15 and 16 year olds like me are having sex. I think feelings are never discussed and that's a problem.
—A teenager from Brooklyn

Safer sex is more than simply knowing how to correctly put on a condom. It is more than being able to recite the four body fluids that carry and transmit HIV. It is more than dental dams, plastic wrap and non-oxynol 9. It is more than mucous membranes, alternatives to sexual intercourse and knowing your partner's HIV status.

Safer sex is feeling safe with the person you are having sex with.

Safer sex is feeling safe enough to stay or safe enough to leave at any moment.

Safer sex is feeling safe enough to communicate everything. If you don't feel comfortable, can you communicate that? If you don't know what your partner intends for you or expects from you, can you find out? If you want to know how often and even with whom they've had sex, do you feel comfortable enough to ask?

Safer sex is caring about yourself so much that no one can make you do anything that you are not 100% comfortable doing.

Safer sex is knowing what you are not 100% comfortable doing.

Safer sex is about knowing yourself so well that you can represent your needs at all times in all situations so that you don't put yourself in a situation of risk.

Safer sex is knowing how to say "no." It's knowing how to say "I don't want to do this." It's knowing how to say, "Yes, there is peer pressure, but no, I'm not playing."

Safer sex is knowing that you are no one's sexual playground to explore and exploit.

Safer sex is knowing that sex is not in your crotch, but in your head and in your heart.

Safer sex is recognizing alcohol and drugs as the intervening variables that affect your better judgment.

Safer sex is being able to listen to conversations about sex without laughing.

Safer sex is being able to look your partner in the face, and not look away.

Safer sex is a vibration, a craving for another person's energy as much as their body.

Safer sex is knowing your partner's last name.

Safer sex is up to you!

In other words, as eleven year old Daniella from Florida puts it, "I want to KNOW you, Boy!"

If you can't talk about sex, then what are you doing having sex? When you are alone with someone in a sexual situation, there's got to be a part of you that silently asks, "Do I feel comfortable here? Am I ready for this? Can I articulate all of my feelings?"

If you think you are old enough, mature enough, comfortable enough, able and ready to have sex, then you better be old enough, mature enough, comfortable enough, able and ready to make your own decisions. And if you are ready to make your own decisions, you better be ready to talk about them. And if you are ready to talk about them, you better be ready to understand the consequences. And if you don't think you are ready to handle the consequences, then you're not ready to have sex.

And if you can't talk about sex with your clothes on, what makes you think it's any easier when your clothes are off?

I don't care about the stigmas. I did when I was your age, and it's one of the reasons I'm infected today. For once, let there be some memory of someone who once said to you, "*It doesn't matter what your sexuality is.*"

I don't care who you have sex with. I care that YOU care who you have sex with.

So if you're going to experiment with sex, try experimenting with love, too. If you can't love your sex partners, at least like them very much. And above all else, try to make each other feel safe. And if you can't even do that, then get out of the bed.

So get honest with yourselves and your partners and start talking.

People just don't talk about sex, period. I mean, people don't even say the word. You know, it may be so taboo to have sex at such young ages, but people don't realize that there are 13 and 14 year-olds having sex at that age. And they attend this camp. They attend any school or camp. And then nobody knows about everything else that goes along with sex, like diseases and HIV, because nobody wants to talk about it. I mean, once you're comfortable talking about it, you know, then you can maybe get others to be comfortable.

Right! The more comfortable you feel talking about sex, the more comfortable your partner will feel talking about sex. If you're not comfortable, that's a start. It's just a matter of being able to say, "I'm not really comfortable talking about this." There's nothing bad about that; it helps, in fact, to break the ice and get your partner talking.

When you tell the truth, others tell the truth. Give people your human-ness. Any opportunity you take to be honest and to reveal yourself in talking with your partner just might make you that much more appealing. AIDS is not just changing our sex lives, but also changing the way we behave in the world so that we respect each other when we have sex.

I know what you're saying and I agree with it, but how do I go to my boyfriend and actually say to him, "These are my fears...?"

You say, "These are my fears..."

It's not easy, I know. Believe me, I know. I'm living with HIV because it was too uncomfortable for me to have that conversation. But let me tell you something, it is infinitely more uncomfortable living with HIV.

Back in December of 1987, I never said, "No, I don't want to do that and I mean it!" or "You must use a condom every time," or "what exactly are we gonna do here," or "how much farther are we gonna go with this," or simply, "I'm scared." More than that, I knew I wasn't safe. I knew I was uncomfortable in my environment, in that apartment. But I thought, "I need to find out about sex. I need to find out about who I am in the world as a sexual being." I was also too embarrassed and ashamed to say "I'm uncomfortable." I didn't know "the right" questions to ask. I was afraid to say "Yes" and I was afraid to say "No." I felt like I should know all those answers and was ashamed that I didn't so I kept my mouth shut. I didn't feel I had any right to say, "I'll do this but not that." Or, "We need to take this whole thing a little slower."

Or simply "Stop!"

There's no difference between you and me except a few years and the fact that I did a few risky things and I got infected. I'm here to tell you what that's about so that you don't do the things I did and put yourselves in a position where you can get into trouble. As one HIV positive friend says, "I'm here to share my experience so you don't experience what I share." Because there is no longer an excuse. No longer can you say, "I didn't know." Or, "I thought it couldn't happen to me." Because if it can happen to me, it can happen to you. And it couldn't have happened to a nicer guy.

Perhaps you can learn through my mistakes. You don't have to know life the way I know life. You can get the same lesson without having the same experience. But then again, this is your life and your learning ground. Think about it. Which is more uncomfortable — a few minutes or maybe even hours of a really difficult conversation which includes your feelings about sex and HIV/AIDS, or living the rest of your life with HIV/AIDS? It's your life. You decide.

What happens when you decide to have that kind of communication? You either have sex or you don't. And you get to know whether or not you even want to have sex with that person. And you get to learn how to talk about sex. And you get to know yourself in a situation where you've never been before. And you get to know your partner better. Communication can do more than just save your life. Communication can create intimacy. It can influence you to look into your partner's eyes and say, "I care about you but I care about myself, too. I'm kind of concerned. How can we help each other through this?"

The excuse "we all make mistakes" doesn't exactly work in this case, you know. You make one mistake and you pay for it for the rest of your life. You can't afford to screw up. And you don't have to be promiscuous, you don't have to be gay, you don't have to be heterosexual, white, black, whatever. You just have to have unsafe sex or share needles. If you put yourself at risk, there's a good chance you will have to face the consequences.

Right. In essence, what we're talking about is much more than AIDS and safer sex. It's about not getting in a car with a drunk person or taking drugs from a friend, or even having friends that do drugs. It's about going home with someone at a party when your inner voice says, "Maybe not", or driving way over the speed limit, or cheating on your boyfriend/girlfriend, or being disrespectful to someone else's property, or simply not liking yourself. It's about life and the way in which you participate in it. It's about self-respect, self-esteem, speaking up for yourselves and taking a stand. It's about peer pressure, using your head and thinking before you take action. It's about discovering what each of your own individual beliefs are and learning to stand behind them. It's about developing a "safety instinct."

And it all starts by asking yourself,

"How does it feel inside?" 🐾

JOSH & ESTHER

Josh was talking to us about love. And his girlfriend. And his lunch. Josh was talking a lot. He was also arguing with Esther, who was sitting next to me. Sarah was sipping her apple juice and smiling. Faith was shaking. Andy was silent.

I was teaching a group of teens who were mentally retarded, or developmentally challenged. In truth, they were teaching me.

Having been informed that their favorite camp activity was the martial arts class, I asked them, "Who can tell me how to defend themselves from physical danger?"

Esther volunteered by raising her elbow in front of her face and saying, "Get away! Just get away!"

"Okay," I goaded. "So how do you defend yourself when you think you are in emotional danger?"

The room was silent. This required further thought.

"I'll make it easier," I said. "How do you defend yourself from something that is dangerous, emotional, and sexual?"

After a bit of explaining to them what I meant, Josh responded, "You listen inside."

And he began to draw for us – a ladder. His "safety ladder," as he called it, was a way of recognizing and protecting one's personal boundaries from physical harm in a sexual encounter. On the first rung, we agreed to place the act of holding hands. On the second, we added the act of putting an arm around another person's shoulder.

"How do you know how far to go?" I asked.

"You need to know the person," someone responded. "You need to feel comfortable with them."

"But what does feeling comfortable feel like?" I prodded.

Once again, they fell silent. They thought long and hard. Finally, Josh said,

"You don't feel butterflies in your stomach."

"You need to take your time. You must go slow. That's important in feeling safe," Esther asserted. Josh added, "If you feel tight inside, that's not good."

Eventually, we agreed if you are ready, you might arrive at the third rung of the ladder which Sara said would be "hugging." Kissing, an embarrassing step for some in the room, was fourth. And fifth, according to Josh, was love.

"Like my girlfriend," he proudly announced. "We've been together for a few months now, and I love her."

"I have a question for you, Josh," I interrupted. "How do you know you love her?"

He sat motionless. His mind was filled with thought while the room waited in silence. Finally, he declared, "I feel a softening in my chest."

When I was growing up, the movie *The Marathon Man* was a big hit. Almost daily, my older brother, Robert, would run around the house haunting me with his favorite line from the film, "Is it safe? Is it safe?" I never knew what it meant in the context of the movie, but it taught me to question how I felt inside. Did my brother know something I didn't? Was I safe in my world? Was I safe with my secrets, my beliefs and my dreams?

One of my teachers once taught me that our bodies respond to feelings and our muscles hold emotions. It follows then that, if attended to, they might inform us of situations of risk. And so one summer day, to a room full of cognitively impaired teenagers, I asked the questions, "Is it safe? How does it feel inside?" Although many of the teens giggled nervously, and some simply didn't respond, Josh and Esther, through their arguing and postulating, described for me something of the emotional processes they go through. Though their cognitive minds may be somewhat impaired, their spirits are extremely developed. Certainly, their insight can be useful to us all.

"I know all that," Josh proudly declared. "It's just that sometimes I don't know how to tell my girlfriend how I really feel."

"Why?" I asked.

"Because I am afraid I might hurt her."

"Aah," I said. "So, everybody, why don't we tell Josh who it is that ends up getting hurt."

And the teens in the room responded with a knowing murmur, "Josh does."

"Josh, repeat after me," I said. "I value myself, and I come first."

———

One young adult that I met this summer pointed out to me that although Josh, Esther and their companions were born with many challenges, they have also come here with many blessings. "Perhaps their souls are so evolved that they have little need for a developed intellect; they respond with their hearts."

If my friend had AIDS

We'd rent movies - not teary ones
And make popcorn - without salt
We'd play wiffle ball - no rules
And rollerblade - no kneepads
We'd lounge on the sofa - without shoes
And watch the Brady Bunch - without cousin Oliver
We'd play in our treehouse - no boys
And build forts - without walls
We'd speak of the future - no fear
And remember the past - no regret

If my friend had AIDS - no cure
She'd have me - without fail

RANA, AGE 16

7

fear

A young man raised his hand during one of my HIV/AIDS support group meetings.

"When I first came to this room a year ago," he shared, "I was newly diagnosed with AIDS, and I remember looking around and asking 'How am I going to find the courage to go on?'

I still haven't found it," he continued. "But the difference is that now I know courage exists."

—*A share at one of my HIV support groups*

How many people in this dining hall know someone who is HIV+ or has AIDS?

(About 50 respond, out of a room filled with 150 teens.)

How do you behave around them? Are you afraid of them or do you treat them differently?

I don't keep my distance, but I'm more conscious of them in the room.

Um, our family has a friend who has HIV, but not AIDS. And at first, when I knew him, I didn't even know, and then my mom told me, and I was like, "Oh, well, it doesn't matter." You couldn't tell.

Do you think you could be a friend of someone who is HIV+?

Um, one of my friends has AIDS and he's had it for a few years. He's my age, fifteen. And I've known that for a long time. And the only thing that I have to be careful of is not touching his blood. So I'm not afraid of him.

Anyone else?

I would keep a distance. I can't help it.

Why?

I'm concerned about getting AIDS.

...of getting infected by being near them?

I just don't feel comfortable around them.

What do you think this distance thing is about? It all comes down to one word.

Fear.

What are we really afraid of?

Getting close to somebody that may die. Losing somebody.

And what happens when we're afraid of people? What do we do?

We stay away from them.

We stay away from them because we don't want anything to happen to us, right? And what happens with that fear? We stay farther and farther away until we realize that we're shutting people

37

out. Yet it's that fear that could hurt us in the end. I once met a girl who said, "If teenagers are afraid of talking about AIDS, then they're the ones at risk."

I know this is kind of difficult to listen to and probably even more difficult to talk about. But there's somebody in this dining hall that may have gotten infected this summer. There's somebody sitting here that may get infected this coming year. I want that person to hear what I have to say and I want the rest of you to know how to handle it if it happens to them or if it happens to you. So listen to what's going on inside yourselves. Why don't you want to hear this?

If you think that some of the things that I am telling you today don't apply to your life right now, that's okay. I'm not here to insult you. But keep your ears open if you can, because one day, I promise you, there will be people in your lives that need to hear this, and you can teach them. You have the power to save lives.

Educating others is the best way to empower yourselves. So listen up...

We've got to find a way to deal with our fear of each other and our fear of AIDS. Where does the fear come from? What purpose can it serve us? In this room is the antidote for some of the fear. It has to do with perception and using our minds. More importantly, it involves using our hearts. The real answer is in communication: in talking to each other and telling the truth, really communicating your sexuality, your needs, your desires and fears to the people that are around you - especially those people you're planning to have sex with. Learn how to deal with each other. I'm talking about connection.

None of you have to go through this life alone.

Hold on to the thought: "We are the same. And because I care, I am going to try to make a difference." It's easier than you think. When you take action and get motivated your fear begins to move away. When you're afraid and discouraged, educate and empower.

How have you been able to get the idea of fear out of your mind?

By admitting I am afraid. We must not be afraid to admit that we're afraid. I start by telling the truth in front of all of you here. Sometimes I get scared. See, I am just like you. If I look at it rather than try to push it away, at least I can say, "Well, that's a part of my human-ness." One of the ways I deal with it is by feeling it, or trying to, anyway.

I always believed that I was only afraid of very few things in life. But after HIV, I see that I have lots of fear and that's okay. I see how I have judged myself for my fear, as if I *was* my fear, instead of remembering it's just visiting me. In fact, I see now that it's more courageous to feel the fear than to believe that it's not there. Just think to yourself, "Fear is visiting me right now. I am in an adrenalized state." Over all, this feeling is about aliveness.

I remember a night a few years ago when I had so much fear of AIDS. I had just watched a horror film and when I turned off the television I started thinking about my life and my death. I was literally on my knees facing my bed, and my hands were shaking so fast that I had to grab onto the bedspread in order to stop them from moving. Finally, I got up off the floor, turned on the lights and walked over to the mirror because I wanted to see what fear looked like on me. I stared and stared at my face in the mirror until I stopped shaking. Somehow looking at myself and being present through the fear helped me to transform it - I was holding it rather than resisting it.

Sometimes fear happens when you are coming out of the dark. Only when you wake up from your nightmares do you scream and shake, when it's safe to feel the fear. I guarantee you, if you try to work with it eventually you will do something to move out of it. You will find a way to motivate yourself and grow from it because you won't want to feel it again. And the next time, you will be a little more familiar with yourself in a state of fear.

I am shit afraid of AIDS.

Beyond the fact of safer sex. Just the actual fact that it's in this world and that it's here, it's living. What advice can you give me to deal with this? There is that burden and that heartache in my soul. Do you feel it too? Do you feel pain? Do you feel joy? Do you feel inspiration? How does anyone, whether they are HIV positive or negative deal with this situation?

You don't know that you can get through a crisis until you get through a crisis. Actually getting through the trauma of being told I was infected taught me how to get through the next difficult experience and somehow I've arrived here today in front of all of you.

Think about the times in your lives when you had to get through a difficult situation. It could have been something as simple as having bad skin or something more difficult like your parents breaking up. Or someone you love dying in a car accident. Or maybe you know someone who has anorexia or bulimia or who may have been abused by family or picked on by friends. Maybe you know someone who committed suicide, or tried to, or is overweight, or has no friends ... a crisis. Whatever it is - it's a crisis. You get through it. Every day. Think about your lives. Think about how you've survived so far.

Realize that you're all stronger than you think you are.

Knowing that I'm not the only one who is afraid of AIDS is also something to think about. There are a lot of people in the world who are dealing with it. It helps just knowing that we are all in this together. We are all frightened.

Think for a second. All of you in this room — think. Who are my allies? Who are those people that I can turn to in a situation of crisis? Who can I talk to about my problems and feelings? Who in my life can I fail or fall apart in front of? Who wouldn't judge me or make fun of me? Who would forgive me? Who can I experience the unknown with? Who would that person be? This is how it starts. You start by building up your support network.

Who can you trust to show the parts of yourself that you don't even want to show yourself? Who can you turn to and say, "This is who I am and I never knew it until I showed it to you." Because true intimacy is not just sharing your secrets and stories with someone. True intimacy is revealing parts of yourself *to* yourself in the presence of another.

In this room is the help you need.
We've taught each other about AIDS.
More importantly, we've taught each other
about the love we already have inside for
each other. This is a way of changing AIDS.
It exists in the way we hold faith. It's in the
way we look at AIDS — from fear, or as
you said, "shit fear", (the room laughs)...to laughter. 🐝

LAURA

"Just be careful of the blonde-haired girl in the front row. She might be a little difficult."

The blonde-haired girl in the front row talks out of turn and has trouble listening quietly. She raises her hand a lot and laughs out loud for no apparent reason. And she doesn't speak clearly. The blonde-haired girl in the front row suffered neurological damage to her brain after a car accident last year.

"I just want you to be aware," her teacher told me before my lecture. "You never know what she's going to say."

I was sitting on a stage in front of four hundred teenagers. I was challenging their opinions by asking a lot of questions. And I was watching out for Laura.

"Who can tell me why teenagers have unsafe sex?" I asked.

I looked around the room and waited, but no one raised their hand. Except for Laura.

I ignored her hand and answered my own question, pontificating and theorizing until I felt it was safe to ask another question. "Does anyone want to share with me what it's like to know someone who has died of AIDS?"

Again I looked around the room and waited, but no one raised their hand. Except for Laura.

I fumbled my way out of calling on her by recounting some of my own experiences but started to get mischievous about this situation. So after a little while, I looked in Laura's direction and asked, "Who here can tell me the exposed mucous membrane in the body most vulnerable to HIV infection, where the blood vessels are closest to the surface of the skin?"

Laura raised her hand.

I was scared of this blonde-haired girl in the front row. I didn't understand her and wasn't sure what would come out of her mouth. I was afraid that she would destroy the mood I had been trying to establish and steal my control of the room.

But I was also a little bit curious about her. What was she thinking?
What was going on in her mind as she sat through my lecture?

A little later on, an HIV positive friend who had been teaching with me spoke to
the room. "This is a question I've been dying to ask for a long time," Bob began.
"Suppose you were dating someone, and you began to care for each other very much
and you wanted to become more intimate with them. Then they told you that they
were HIV positive. What would you do?"

The students were quiet. Some rustled in their seats.
Some looked around at each other.

But Laura raised her hand. And Bob called on her to speak.

Her words came out slowly and painfully, devoid of any deliberate inflection or
emotion. Her face contorted as she strained to form each syllable with incredible
humility and utter plainness. The single sentence she delivered seemed like minutes
to create, and the anticipation for each word drew me closer to her. And with a final
syllable, she had breached the distance I had securely positioned between us.

> "If ... I ... really ... cared ... for ... him ...
> ... it ... wouldn't ... matter."

We sat in silence. Four hundred teens, Bob and I. Just breathing.
Listening to the silent echo of her words. Suddenly, punctuating the serenity
of the moment, the bell rang.

And I thought to myself, "See...that's God. I just heard God say, 'Amen, Laura. Amen.'"

I do not have much money, so

I will give you my time
I will talk for you
I will walk for you

I do not have the knowledge to cure you, so
I will give you my time
I will visit when you're lonely
I will hug you when you're frightened

I do not have the answers, so
I will give you my time
I will listen when you're angry
I will hold you when you cry

I do not have the heart to leave, so
I will give you my time
I will stay when you need me to
I will give you my time

SARAH, AGE 14

8

testing

A thirteen year-old girl asked my favorite question. "What is the one thing you want to hear
from someone after you tell them that you are HIV+?" I was stunned by her sensitivity and
was caught by surprise. Finally, after a long silence, I answered. "What can I do to help?"

—*A camper in Pennsylvania*

Tell me why a group of teenagers would sign up for an AIDS lecture on a summer Saturday morning? What brought you here?

Because AIDS seems like one of the most important topics now. Because we are teenagers and sex is a main factor in our lives. And 'cause AIDS is such a huge problem and causing people to get ill and die just because they are having sex.

I think you could never be educated enough about it. In my health class, we did a whole three days on AIDS. But all you heard were the statistics and I figured that this workshop would be a lot more educational.

This is what I simply don't understand. In high school, you have pre-calc or chemistry or social studies every day. Why don't you have AIDS education every day? Or classes in self-esteem and self-confidence and learning refusal skills — every day?

I've heard other speakers on AIDS and it seems like everybody's story is totally different about what happened to them. I think it's important to hear all the different stories because it didn't just happen to one life.

What would you like to know about my story?

What was it like to tell your parents?

All I will say is that I never truly knew the color of my mother's eyes, until I saw them the moment I told her.

What made you decide to get tested and what was it like?

I got tested because I knew that I was playing with fire. I knew I was fooling around without a condom. I also got an acute onset, the flu-like symptoms that sometimes come when your bloodstream is converting from negative to positive. Since my sex partner told me he was born with syphilis, I thought maybe it was that. I was praying it was. Can you imagine praying for syphilis? Think about it for a second. Because if it wasn't that, then maybe it was the onset of HIV infection.

What was your first reaction when you found out?

I was in a clinic in New York City and it was 10:00 in the morning. Someone called my number, 224, ironically my homeroom number from high school. I went to the next waiting room. I sat there and waited. I watched a tall man disappear into one office, get a folder which I believed to be mine, then disappear into another office. Back and forth, back and forth, from office to office, with this folder in his hand. After a while, I started to worry, until he finally called me in.

With the folder now open, he was leaning against the front of a grey metal desk. It was the kind my grade school teachers had, and I instantly remembered being back in fifth grade getting caught picking at the scotch tape stuck to the side of Mr. Campbell's desk. I knew it was a "wrong thing to do" but I couldn't help breaking the rules...just this once.

"My name is Larry," he said. His voice brought me back into the room. He looked down at the papers in the folder and back up at me and then down again. And I thought, "I'm so vulnerable in this moment. This moment is lasting forever. And there's nothing I can do about it. I feel short. I feel young. I feel afraid. He can change my life forever with one word: yes or no, positive or negative. This man whom I've never seen before may never leave my memory." And as I'm waiting for that moment to hit me, I noticed how he was just leaning there, his body weighted against the edge of the desk, with one arm behind him, this stranger holding my future in the folder in his hand.

"Okay," he said. Yet even during the pronunciation of that one small word I was still aware of the cruelty of time and how it seemed to keep stretching. "Well, here are the results. And... I'm... sorry... it's positive... but before you..."

And in the next moments between the words "it's positive" and "but before you...," I lived an entire lifetime.

The room went white. My life went white. Everything was stark and I thought, "OK, we're gonna just survive here. We're gonna just stay alive. We're gonna just do this one day at a time, one minute at a time, one millisecond at a time."

Then I saw a picture in my mind of my mother wiping a brown dresser with a white rag. It was my childhood bedroom at home on a Sunday morning, and I was just returning from Hebrew School. And everything on that dresser was gone. Wiped away. She was wiping everything away.

The second thing I saw was my mother in the room standing behind me but facing the other way. In the movie in my mind, with the same white rag, she was wiping the windowsill in the room in that clinic, looking out onto the drug-infested streets of 9th Avenue. And I realize now the connection: the end of innocence, the abolishment of my childhood.

The third thought was whether I would ever be able to have children of my own, and the dangers involved in impregnating a woman.

The fourth thought I had was of my father and the time when I was a little boy on Christmas break from grade school. My father took me to his school where he used to teach. We were going to spray paint some weights in the gym but I couldn't get the paint can to spray. So like any normal, curious and not careful nine year-old, I looked at the nozzle and pressed down on it and sure enough it was working. My father rushed me to the bathroom and washed all the yellow paint out of my eye. First, I was scared because he was scared. And then I relaxed because he relaxed. He took care of it as fathers are supposed to do, as we expect them to do. And in this moment, in the fourth millisecond after I heard, "I'm sorry...it's positive," I saw my father, back when I was nine years old, and I heard him say to me, "I'm sorry, Scotty. This time I can't get you out of this. I can't take this one away."

My mind came back to the room when I heard the counselor say to me, "...but before you leave here today, I want to give you some phone numbers to call. I don't ever want to see your face again. You'll be fine. You're young and strong and healthy. You should have no problems."

When you are in crisis, time slows down and moments move in slow motion. You become aware of every single thought behind every single thought. Sometimes I think that's actually what is meant by "living in the moment," being completely aware of where you are and what you are experiencing. My entire life was in front of me and behind me and all these pictures and images were playing on the screen in my mind, a millisecond at a time. You've heard the expression, "I saw my whole life pass before my eyes." Well, I saw my whole future pass before my eyes and I wanted it more than ever before.

Did you ever doubt God?

My brother, Norman, once said to me: "Scotty, everybody loses God. We find Him when we need Him." When I heard the words "I'm sorry, it's positive...," I needed God then. I knew that God probably had something to say to me. And I was ready to listen.

It seems to me that in order to *doubt* God you must first believe in God. Remember that while part of you is doubting, there's that other part that is believing. And if you can just witness that, in part, you are still believing...you're not totally doubting, are you? Think about it.

My goals and dreams and aspirations are the same as yours. I still want the same things you want, happiness, love, friendship, a long life and a lot of attention. But knowing that I'm HIV positive is important too because I can watch my bloodwork closely, measure the level of stress in my life, make the necessary changes, try different kinds of therapies and most of all, go after my dreams. There's work to be done. So I think it was a good thing that I got tested.

Now should *you* get tested? Well, that's your choice. But think about it before you do. If you get tested and the results are positive, what would you do? Where would you go? Would you be okay not knowing? All I can tell you is that I'm glad I know. Because if I didn't know that I was infected, I would never be the person I am today — able to just be here in front of you.

So what did that experience teach me? It taught me that we all have a lifetime, we just don't know how long that lifetime will be. And it taught me that life is made up of moments that never leave us; that in this moment, everything exists. We don't know what the next moment is, so this one is the most important. And what is the most important thing about this moment? It has something to do with support, compassion, caring and love. I'm no different than any of you. I'm really not. It's just that I have a daily reminder that this day is the only day. And as a result, what matters most is what happens right here and right now. All of you in this room. ❧

NICK

"I hear your name is Nick," I gently said to a young teenager crying on the bleachers. He was sitting by himself at the back of the gym after my lecture. He was sobbing uncontrollably.

I climbed up next to him and sat motionless for a few brief moments as I listened to him weep. Eventually, I encroached upon his private space by nudging my elbow into his side and sighing semi-audibly. Tenderly, I said, "Nick?"

In between his sobs, he said, "Uh-huh."

I reached across him to rest my arm on his tiny shoulder. "You don't have to tell me anything. I just want to sit here while you cry. Is that okay with you?"

Again, he grunted. "Uh-huh."

"But if you wanted to talk, then..."

"There's a lot of people dying in my life right now" he blurted. "My aunt died of cancer and my grandfather died of cancer and I miss them."

I thought about this for a moment. "What do you miss most about your grandpa, Nick?" I asked.

"Golfing. He used to take me golfing. He was my best friend."

"I'll bet he was really proud to have you for a grandson."

"Uh-huh," he replied.

And after I exchanged his crumpled ball of used tissues for some clean ones, I asked him, "Nick, do you ever...talk to him?"

"Uh-huh. All the time. I really believe in that kind of stuff."

"What do you tell him?" I prompted.

"I tell him I miss him," he said, ignoring the tissues as he wiped his nose with the bottom of his T-shirt.

We sat in silence for a while longer.

"I can't stop crying," he lamented, speaking through his shirt.

"So don't," I said. "Just keep crying until you have no more tears left to cry. And then, Nick...then, cry some more."

"Uh-huh," he answered. "That's how I feel about it."

We sat some more. I listened as he cried.

"Nick?" I asked. "Is there anything that you haven't done this summer that you'd like to do?"

"Uh-huh," he answered, finally lifting up his head so that I could see part of his tear-streaked face. "I'd like to perfect my jump shot in basketball."

"Then why don't you make that your goal for the summer?" I suggested. "And when you achieve it, know that your grandfather will be watching. But don't do it just for him. You must do it for yourself."

"Uh-huh," he grunted. And as he turned his whole diminutive body towards me, he asked, "Um, if I write to you, will you write me back?"

I looked fully into his face now and saw for the first time who it was I had been sitting with and talking to. And smiling down on him, I answered.

"Uh-huh."

I pray that love is enough

I pray that I remember smiles like I remember the sun
I pray for sacred scenes
Like falling into love and never falling out
Laughter with my mother
Holding open doors for strangers

I know that death is for all
And I pray that in its face we can hold hands
And say yes to life

GOWRI, AGE 18

9

death

In the hospital...I got that this is the miracle. This is the way God does it. Why question His way? And once I realized that, suddenly the hospital room wasn't the hospital room anymore. And the elevator door wasn't the elevator door. It was the process of life. And all I could say was "Thank You." That's all there is to say. "Thank you for the experience."

—Richard 1959 - 1994

I have a document on my computer at home entitled "Deaths," with the names and dates of friends that have died from AIDS. So far, there are over one hundred and twenty-five names on that list. My date book is filled with more deathdays than birthdays; it's like a holocaust in my soul. People die of AIDS all the time and if you don't know about it because it's not a part of your immediate world, I am here to tell you that it's a part of someone else's. It is real.

Has anybody here ever been in the hospital when someone was dying?

I have. It's very depressing. You don't know what to say. You have mixed feelings. My grandma died just recently, and I was there watching her. It's like I felt glad it wasn't me, but also sad that it was her, you know? And like, mixed up in a lot of different ways.

My uncle died of AIDS. I didn't want to visit him or even talk with him. I was afraid to go to the hospital. I mean, what do you do when you see a person in the hospital that you love and you want to say "how are you" but you know what they're gonna say? Why bother saying "how are you?"

You don't know how they are until you ask. They may surprise you. Ask. Joseph Campbell, the late author and historian, once said, "the privilege of life is being allowed to be who we truly are." I would add, "especially as we're dying."

Does anybody feel like they learned from the people they watched die?

Well, my grandma, when she died, she taught me a lot. I remember she was dying for, like, two straight years in a row and she would try to make me understand. She would tell me, like, "if it happens, it happens. Everybody should die someday."

When we visit people who are dying, we think we're going there to help them, when actually we find they help us.

They touch places inside our hearts that we didn't know needed to be touched. We can discover things just in the way they breathe in and breathe out. I have learned that all you ever need to do when a person is dying is just be there and tell the truth. Just show up and love them — which is the truth.

Yesterday, I was visiting a friend in the hospital with AIDS. He can't see me anymore because he lost his eyesight, but he was excited to hear it was me and said, "Stand up...over here." He reached his arm out and pulled me to his chest and held my head down pretty hard. I kept pulling myself away to give him my hand instead. He'd relax for a minute, then grab at me and pull me down again.

"Help me. Help me," he said. "I have to go."

"Where?"

"To the white room," he said.

"Where's the white room?" I asked.

"It's over there...in the next room. How do I get there?"

"Close your eyes," I answered. "Relax. There's no rush. You'll get there."

All I could do was create and hold a space for him to do it his way, in his time.

And love him.

How about you? Aren't you half-scared that you might die?

Yes, but let me ask you something. Aren't you half-scared that you might die? I am no different from any of you. It's something else we all have in common. We're all gonna die.

I am afraid when you talk like this. The thought of me not being around tomorrow scares the hell out of me. I have not made up my mind to die. It might sound stupid, but I'm serious.

It doesn't sound stupid at all. We all think about death. Sometimes we even sit down and cry about it. Certainly, we all have something to say about it.

I'm saying, how do you feel knowing that you are HIV positive and that somewhere down the line you may not make it to 35. I would be pissed to shit. Still in my mind, although I know I have to die, I'm not ready. I don't want to die now.

Sometimes I think that I'll be ready for it when it comes. And sometimes, like today, I'm not. Sometimes, I live fully in the moment and other times I live so fully that it's stressful trying to make every moment matter, not letting a minute go by without filling it with awareness and alertness. But I've come to the understanding that, yes, I am going to die. I don't know if it's going to be from AIDS or from something else. But it's going to be on a day of a week of a month of a year in my life. My feelings about life and death may seem urgent and more pressing because I'm looking at these issues almost daily, but it's the same for you. We all get to know the feelings associated with death because it is something we all get to do. These are just days, a bunch of days strung together. The real question is, what are you going to do with yourselves in the meantime?

Why bother trying to solve death? I mean, can we even solve life?

These many years have taught me many things. I have learned how to help my friends recover and how to help my friends die. We are learning together that sometimes death is a gift in that it teaches us something more about life. Ultimately, I am no better, no stronger, and no more special in the eyes of God than those who have gone before me.

If I were to die of AIDS in the next few years and you were to hear about it, I don't want you all to think that we failed. Yes, I pray that there is a medical cure that eradicates the virus from existence. But let's talk about a cure as a shift in the way that we look at this so that as people continue to die of AIDS, and maybe myself included, our lives will not have been failures. I make my life worthwhile because this moment and the next matter to me.

Sometimes I am so scared of dying - like my life is only leading towards death. The only way I can solve that fear is to learn to totally love my friends and my life, each day. I mean, then, when I die, I will know that the love I've felt will last into eternity. ✶

**Lying in my hospital bed, looking at the ceiling,
I realized, it's just me and God. That's all it is.
That's what did it for me. I just prayed each night
for Him to just be with me. That's all. Just be with me.
And give me peace and take the pain. That's all.
It's just life. We know that. And yeah I have fear.
I'd lay there and think, this is it. So this is it. And then
I'd think, what is it? It's just life.**

—*Curtis, 1960-1993*

JENNIFER

Tonight, some older campers were asked to work on a project for the charity of their choice. They decided to create a few panels to add to the Names Project AIDS Memorial Quilt.

I explained to them that the Quilt, made up of thousands of fabric panels, is an ongoing memorial and visual reminder of lives lost by AIDS. I recounted the day I first saw it laid out in its entirety on the Mall in Washington, D.C.

"Someone was reading names," I explained. "...thousands of names of people that died of AIDS, each one read aloud, with weighted sentiment. And as I placed my foot onto the grass on the Mall — crossing the boundary from bystander to participant on this day of commemoration, on this day of tribute — I heard the reader pronounce, out of thousands on the list, the name of my dear friend, Steven, whose panel I had come to see."

After speaking to the campers, I enlisted without much trouble twenty open-hearted volunteers. Together we set out to make a panel for Jennifer, my best friend, who died of AIDS at the age of twenty-seven.

I told them a little about the day she and I met. We were at a People With AIDS workshop six months after I found out my HIV status. I instantly noticed her in the crowd of PWA's because of our "sameness." Up till then, I didn't believe there were actually people so much like myself that were infected. She was the first ally in my new world, my first HIV positive friend...and one of the first to die.

The topic of the workshop on the morning we met was loveless sex, and the room was arguing that any kind of disease of the spirit starts with a lack of love. Jennifer raised her hand.

"I need some help with what I'm feeling right now," she said. "I got infected with HIV from a man I met one weekend on a ski trip when I was in college," I recall her tearfully saying. "...and the thing that hurts the most is that it wasn't loving."

Then I showed the campers the friendship ring she gave me on that very day, which I wear still. Two circles of silver, ever intertwined. "The rules of giving," she explained to me, "are that whatever is given to you must be given away to someone else someday. We only borrow the gifts that are given us. Love stays, but even that is a gift that needs to be given away."

I told them a little about how she loved to giggle and dance. "At times," I said, "we'd be dancing together, and we couldn't look into each other's eyes without laughing wildly until one of us would have to leave the room. And usually it was Jennifer."

And I told them how her last words, "I love you, too," were spoken only to me.

Then they went to work on her panel. They created, in a matter of three hours, a true and genuine representation of what Jennifer-meant to me. One camper named Marc drew a picture in magic marker that looked just like her, laughing and dancing, with wings on her feet.

It was utterly astonishing to watch the process: the summoning of her likeness and energy out of me, and woven into the felt and fabric on the floor before us. They designed and drew, stenciled and sewed. They coordinated and created, dominated and surrendered. Each assigned themselves a task: cutting, choosing colors, imagining, watching, working together.

"I drew from your memories," Katherine said to me. "You inspired me when you told your heartwarming stories and made the tears fall from my eyes. Before you, I had never met anyone who was HIV positive. You inspired me with your energy and vitality."

When midnight arrived with a sudden summer storm, we were a collection of campers - turned artists - turned partners - gathered in a huge barn. Standing in a circle, shouldered by one another, we looked down on the work we had done. We stared in hushed wonder at how a sheet and scissors and some string could suddenly and silently command our innermost attention.

After a while, when the rain had shifted, leaving August's evening dust in the air, I told them the story of the night Jennifer died.

"She was in bed. And alone," I began. "I was hurt to see how sick and in pain and alone she seemed."

"Hi," she said. But that was all she would offer. She had a lot of pain that night, especially in her chest and the area behind her ribs. She kept screaming, "Oh shit...

it hurts, it hurts."

"How do you do it, Jenn?" I thought to myself. "You've been through so much. So much suffering."

I went around to the other side of the bed where her head was turned toward the window, knelt down on my knees and looked into her eyes. "I know it hurts Jenn. I can see you're in pain. It hurts a lot, doesn't it?"

"Yes."

There I was, on my knees, on the floor of this empty room in the hospital, staring straight into her eyes. She soaked in my gaze; she locked it in place. I wanted to look away because it lasted for so long, but I didn't dare. I knew she needed my eyes then. I didn't see magic or angels or God. But I did feel warmth, and some fear, and a searching for something to hold on to. Mostly, though, I felt the fullness of her gaze, the deep and meaningful silence of her stare. And her pain stopped. I could see it in her face. I could hear it in her breathing. I could feel it in the room.

"I am ever amazed at the power of friendship," I told the campers.

I talked to the youngsters about the songs her mom and aunt softly sang to her later that night, while sitting on her bed. "A - You're Adorable, B - You're so Beautiful..." And then, "Thank Heaven For Little Girls."

All this time, Jennifer had been carrying on an inner dialogue. She kept saying, "Uh-huh, yeah, uh-huh." So we'd repeat it. I thought that maybe she was trying to communicate with us, showing us she's alive. Maybe it was something else. All that mattered, though, was helping her in any way I could - stroking her hair, smiling at her and making her giggle, which until tonight was always so easy.

I noticed how blessed I was to have these final moments. I remembered us, Jennifer and I, having breakfasts at the diner and waving goodbye at the bus stop. "You did good, girl," I muttered to myself. "You really did it! And I'm so proud." We prayed for this, for some sort of peace at the end of our mortal campaign. I suppose we prayed for a beautiful "deathness" in all our entreaties for a life fulfilled.

And now, standing in a circle inside a rain-washed barn, I shared with the young campers my experience five years later as I stood in front of Jennifer's grave. I had come to offer a mourner's Kaddish, a Jewish prayer to honor her memory. I stood beneath the weeping willow beside her headstone, and as a soft wind stirred and a single willow branch tapped on my shoulder, I remembered some of Jennifer's last words.

"In those final days," I revealed, "a rabbi came to see her. He asked her if she believed that anything continues after life." Her answer, now stenciled and sewed into the cloth on the floor before us was, "Of course there's more when we die. Where else would music go?"

The nights here at camp are filled with motion. Crickets scrape incessantly, moths pull themselves away from wooden walls, and teenagers begin their search within. And on this special Tuesday night, while the twelve year-old boys, in the darkness of their cabin, in their bunk beds, were noiselessly plotting their midnight assault strategy on the girls' bunk across the pebbled path, a handful of older teens were beginning to grasp the grace that enters when the spirit softens and the willingness to work together becomes the highest goal.

The next day, the huge barn was flooded from the heavy rains the night before, and the ink on the cloth panel smudged like a rainbow-colored oil streak. I was upset until one camper reminded me to consider the positive in every situation.

"We all had so much to do with the quilt," she said reassuringly. "Maybe the flood was Jennifer's way to add her own little touch. And look at the picture we drew of her. She's still smiling."

I hope that my life will not change from this moment
All my friends gathered together
Working together
For I consider my friends as part of my family

Every time I go over a train track
Or through a yellow light
When it is 11:11
Or my recent birthday
I wish for my life to stay the same

Love is the most important thing
The main thing in my life will be love
Because without love there is no life

JEREMY, AGE 18

IO

suicide

A ten year-old girl approached me on the campgrounds as she was running to play. "Just one question," she said. "Do you blame yourself for getting infected?" I took a deep a breath and began to pull together all the conflicted thoughts in my mind, wondering how to answer her sensitive question, when before I could utter a single word, she looked straight into my eyes and said with a smile,

"...because you better not!"
—A camper in North Carolina

Did you ever want to die? Did you not want to go through all this?

I get that question all the time and I always answer with the same story from my favorite movie, "The Secret Garden." Colin is a wheelchair-bound boy who has never been outdoors. "I can't breathe the air outside. It'll kill me," he tells his young cousin Mary. "Everyone says I'm dying."

Mary says, "Well, if everyone said that about me, I just wouldn't do it."

If someone were to tell me tomorrow, "You are HIV-positive", I think I would go crazy. I don't know what would happen to me.

You *think* you think you'd go crazy, but you probably wouldn't. I thought I'd go crazy, too. The minute before the test results were given to me, I thought the same thing. A minute later, I didn't go crazy. I survived. It's amazing how you survive when you have to. You come through when you're challenged by adversity. You just adjust. And you become stronger.

You get your test results back, and one of the things you realize is that life is more important to you than ever before. When you can see that the stakes are high enough, suddenly life becomes worthwhile. Sometimes, when the control is taken out of your hands, you want it back and you find yourself saying, "I want to live more than ever." You want to regain control of your destiny. AIDS makes you more aware of your life wish.

I don't know. If I was faced with that dilemma every day, living with AIDS or killing myself, I don't know if I could decide to just live with it.

Aah. But you are faced with dilemmas every day. Every day of your life you are faced with some sort of crisis and the choice of how to deal with it is entirely up to you. Yet you seem to keep choosing to live. In fact, you got up this morning and came here and have decided to share some of yourself with us. Notice that and give yourself credit. Look, we're all living with AIDS. Whether we're HIV positive or HIV negative, it's in our lives. It's in our world. It's in this room right now. Acknowledge for yourselves that you're doing a pretty good job of living with it.

I know eight teenagers who have killed themselves, including the star athlete in my school.

That's hard to hear. It makes me think of what a person with AIDS once said in a support group. "I feel like every cell in my body has a tear to shed." Sadness and pain are some of the things that make you important to this world. Feel them. Find the courage to work through them. It's what makes a room full of people turn their heads to you in silence, because they know you understand them.

I was watching a popular television show one night, and I heard the line, "You know there's no future in dating someone who is HIV+." Later that evening, on the eleven o'clock news, I saw a teenager being interviewed because her best friend had killed herself. Seems she was diagnosed HIV+. Not AIDS. No sickness. No hospitalization. Just HIV. And she killed herself. Now I don't know any of the reasons she did that, but I'll give you some of the ones I came up with. In our society we don't take enough care of each other by protecting authenticity, presenting the truth of the situation. We create dramas out of things that have no business being sensationalized. We don't talk about the other part of AIDS - the blessings of AIDS.

It is really important that we present the topic of AIDS truthfully, as it really is. That includes a lot of faith, a lot of hope and a lot of love. Support. Religion. Family. Friends. Sharing. Caring. Compassion. Tolerance. Prayer. They're a part of AIDS, too.

Do you understand what I am saying? Because if a teenager finds out they are positive, and all they hear about is the bad news, what reason would they have not to kill themselves?

I'm glad I didn't want to kill myself. Because if I had, I wouldn't have learned all the lessons about myself and life that I have learned over all these years. I wouldn't have become the man that I have become, or met the people that I have met and had the joy and felt the love and taken the opportunities to make life important. Like my friend, Edgardo, said to me the night before he died: "Scott! Get a life!"

If I were to be told tomorrow that I'm HIV positive, what can you tell me that you would want me to remember?

Just...keep...breathing. And what I mean by that is two different things. First, just get through the moment. Inhale and exhale and love each breath that takes you to the next one. Just breathe and get through it because the thoughts will come, the feelings will come, and the energy will come. Just keep breathing. And second, don't kill yourself. Stay here. Stay with the program. Stay alive.

CAREY

Carey was screaming at me from the back of the rec hall, in a crowd of about two hundred teens.

"My mom sat me down a while ago and said, 'Carey, I'm so sorry that you have to live in a world where this is a problem.' You know... it makes me so angry that I have to live in a world like this. Why can't it be in the 50's or 60's when 'Donna Reed' and 'Leave It To Beaver' came on t.v. and that was the lifestyle? And it makes me so angry and so sad to see you up here educating us instead of sitting here and listening with all of us on how to prevent it. Doesn't it make you so mad that you could have... I mean... I know you're trying your hardest to sit people down and say, 'Look, I've made this mistake and I'm learning and I'm proud of myself now' but I just can't even imagine...I'm sitting here thinking, 'What are my kids gonna do?' I'm in this world right now, and if this is a problem today, what's it gonna be like in ten years when I'm already having my children?"

"You're name is Carey, right? Okay Carey, here's my answer. Listen carefully... 'cause here it is.

Love.

I promise you, as sure as I'm standing up here in front of you, healthy as I've ever been, healthier in fact than I was before I got infected...love will get you through. I'm not that afraid. I am with you and you are with each other. And one day, when you have kids of your own, you will make it through. You will have God on your side. When we leave the moment that we're in and start worrying about what's going to happen in the future, we leave where we are right now and right now has everything we need. I'm with you and I'm not afraid. I'm not. I'm not even angry anymore. Because I'm with you. I have passion. I sing. I fight. I play. I never stop talking. I deal. And Carey... I love. And then I go to bed at night, and I get up the next morning and I realize, 'You know what? I made it through.' And so will you. And so will you. And so will you. Do you know what I'm saying?"

"No, I don't! You don't know what's gonna happen tomorrow! You don't know that something's gonna happen to you or me. I don't want to keep taking up all your

time, but I've never met anyone with HIV before and I'm sitting here, facing you and I'm so angry at the world!"

"Good! It's all good! But also think about this: it's not such a bad world. It's not. It's just the world. We think it's so bad, but it's just what we're given. And if you can learn to forgive, learn to surrender, learn to understand and have tolerance for people's differences, never forgetting to sing and fight and play, you'll get up tomorrow morning and you'll get through."

"But tolerance isn't enough! Like...don't you get that? I have diabetes, you know. And I'm waiting for a cure to come. At least there's a remedy. There's insulin to take. There's no cure for AIDS. And I don't want to tolerate that. You know? Why would I put myself in the position to be out to get something else? I've got enough to worry about. Everyone else has enough to worry about. Why...why would anyone not want to care about themselves enough to...like...do you know what I'm trying to say?"

"Absolutely. I couldn't say it better myself, Carey. Why wouldn't you care about your-selves? And when I speak of tolerance, I don't mean to say that we should tolerate the disease and the fact that there's no cure. I'm talking about tolerating each other. That's the love I'm talking about. It's really wise and it's really deep. Give it a chance.

And you're crying, Carey. That's what's wonderful. Do you know why? Because that's all the stuff inside of you saying, 'I want to live! Look at me. I'm Carey...and I want to live!'"

Life is good
But not fair at all

Life is sweet
Yet much too short

Life is what you make of it
Right now and forward

I don't know anyone who has AIDS
If I did
I would make life
with them

JORDAN, AGE 19

I I

heroes

If I grow up, I want to continue to love, no matter how much pain comes along with it.

—*Orit, Age 15*

By a show of hands, how many of you in this room know somebody who is living with HIV?

That's about one quarter of you. Okay, I want all of you to put your hands up. Everybody put your hands in the air. C'mon. All of you. Because all of you know somebody living with HIV.

I am.

(Silence)

Everybody take a deep breath with me...and another one. Now this time make a sound as you exhale...let out a sigh. I want to hear a really deep and really long sigh.

Okay. Now let me just look at you. Let me see who it is I've been given the honor to stand in front of and learn from tonight. Just sit there and show me who you are.

The most important thing I can teach you tonight about HIV/AIDS is simply this:

Learn how to open your mouths and say:

> **"I like myself."**
>
> **"I like myself, therefore, I will not harm myself."**
>
> **"I like myself, therefore, I will not let somebody harm me."**
>
> **"I like myself, therefore, I will not do IV drugs."**
>
> **"I like myself, therefore, I will not have sex if I am not ready."**
>
> **"I like myself, therefore, I will not have sex without a condom."**
>
> **"I like myself, therefore, I will not put myself at risk."**
>
> **"I like myself, therefore, I will not do something stupid!"**

And then, when you are ready, go one step farther and learn to trade the word "like" for "love."

Before I got infected, I didn't know anything about this stuff. I was confused and couldn't speak up on my own behalf. I didn't know how to find out that I was okay exactly as I was. I didn't know how to say, "I have a life worth living. I have a life worth saving."

Sometimes it's so difficult being a teenager that it seems easier just to break the rules and say, "Whatever!" Sometimes it's so difficult being a teenager that it seems easier not to care about the consequences of your actions. And sometimes it's so difficult being a teenager that it seems like no one can possibly ever truly understand you. I salute you for being who you are. I don't think enough people do that. Congratulations. You got out of bed this morning, you laughed and you played, you picked on people and you complained, you ate bad food and you got here. And you'll get up tomorrow morning and do it all over again, and you'll continue to do it every morning because you are heroes.

It's not easy being a teenager today. Salute yourselves. You are all champions. Know that about yourselves. I have spoken to so many of you and what I've learned is that every single one of you counts.

Every single one of you matters. Every single one of you has something to offer this world.

You ache, you cry, and you continue to hope. You have secret feelings and unrevealed needs. You know pain. You know loneliness. You know joy and you know love. You all know something about life. All of you have experienced something which helps you understand the levels of the human condition.

You each have a story to tell. Tell it! Show the world how wonderful you are.

If we all do something little, it turns into something big!

My friend, John, a few months before he died of AIDS, said this to me: "When a tree reaches up to drink in the sun, it doesn't ask if it is deserving." You all deserve to drink in the sun. You all deserve to be heard and to be seen. And you all deserve to be loved. You breathe. You belong. It's enough.

Don't be scared of AIDS. Be smart.

Or as one teenager says, "Think Positive! Stay Negative!" Find out how. Read. Talk. Cry. Call the hotlines and get the facts. Call your friends. Call anybody. Ask. Argue. Educate. Because the more you know, the less you'll fear.

As you go through life, keep remembering that you know about life. Congratulations. You have survived this far, you'll survive even farther. You're going to be great people. This I know.

We misunderstand AIDS. Have I showed you that it's more than just sickness and death and loneliness and punishment and sadness? It's love. Have I showed you that at least a little bit tonight? It's life. It's you.

AIDS is the great equalizer that breaks us down and shows us how much we all have in common: a life worth living. AIDS is the catalyst: the thing that pushes you into full gear. AIDS gives you a kick in the butt and says, "Live now! Make it worthwhile. Show me how much you love life."

Now repeat after me:

I value this day

I value my life

I value your life

I care about my future

I care about you so please care about yourself

And even though I make mistakes, still I try

Look around the room. Some of you are crying. Some of you are hugging. Some of you are yawning. But you're here. You haven't walked out. You showed up and listened and hopefully you're getting something out of it. This, my friends, is what life is all about. Right here. It's the way you wipe your eyes. The way you laugh. The way you hold each other. The way you look after each other and say, "I want you to stay alive. I don't want you to get sick. I don't want you to do something stupid. I don't want you to become infected with HIV. I will look after you. I will make sure of that. And I will make sure of myself."

Remember your feelings tonight. Remember to cherish what's been given you. And always remember that there is hope. ❦

ALISHA

"...the spirit has its own destiny," a counselor says as I approach the flagpole.
I watch as two children release a butterfly from a netted cage into the cool air of
the breaking day. Someone leans over to inform me in a whisper that we are watching a memorial service for the kids that died this year. The crowd, with a muffled
cheer, encourages the child holding the trapped butterfly.

"Keep trying, he'll fly out soon."

It is early morning at a camp for children with cancer and AIDS. Eighty-five youngsters, with life-challenging illnesses, along with their siblings, spend a week together
at the height of summer.

Walking away from the flagpole, a camper named Terry, with her hands fixed in her
back pockets, asked me, "Why are you so alive?"

"What do you mean?" I replied. I think she was referring to my animated behavior
all week. Indeed, I was often singing and dancing.

"I mean were you ever so happy that you were afraid to let yourself feel it for fear
of losing it?"

"I think so," I said, beginning to understand her question. "Sometimes I'm so afraid
to really feel joy. Sometimes, I'm so afraid to surrender to the very next moment
because I'm trying to engrave the immediate one in my memory. But letting go is
only half of it," I said to her. "Letting come must follow."

—

The next day, in music class, I asked the campers to write poems entitled, "If I Could
Ask God One Question." I then read each poem out loud while Doug, the music
counselor, strummed two or three chords on his guitar. Finally, I asked the room to
sing along with me, chanting each child's wishes to their own special melody.

Jon didn't want me to read his poem out loud but he did give permission to have a
song written about it. His request to God was,

"What age will I live till? Because I think it would be cool to live for a long time."

I simply had the whole room sing, "Jon. Jon. You're gonna live forever. Because we love you, Jon."

He was silent and he was still. He listened as the young singers soothingly intoned this mantra. Though his body didn't move, the expression on his face revealed his inner thoughts. He was touched.

Renee, whose leg is in a brace, is little and doesn't like to smile. Renee likes to grade people, mostly with a display of two thumbs down. That's how you know she's paying attention. So on this day, she got a song of her own, using the words from her poem.

> *Thumbs up. Thumbs up. My name is Renee.*
> *Thumbs up. Thumbs up. And here is what I say.*
> *"My question to God may sound silly, but here I go:*
> *You're always over us, do you use the toilet bowl?"*
> *Thumbs up. Thumbs up. My name is Renee.*

Renee was smiling.

Alisha handed me an unfinished poem about her grandparents who died two years ago — unfinished because she stopped in the middle to cry. As I read what she had written, I remembered reading somewhere that "some people only cry when they feel there is hope in sight."

"My question to God. How do you watch over everyone at the same time? How do you give out wishes?"

I asked Doug for some sweet chords and once again closed my eyes.
With the chorus of campers eager to echo, I began to pray.

Oh God, Oh God

It's me again, Alisha

And God, Oh God

It's me again, I need ya

Are you watching over me?

Will you give my wish to me?

'Cause God, Oh God

It's me again, Alisha

Dear Dear Dear Alisha

It's me, it's God, I hear ya

Dear Dear Dear Alisha

It's me, it's God, I'm near ya

And Alisha, just like you

I need you, too

Dear Dear Dear Alisha

Oh God, Oh God

It's me again, Alisha

And God, Oh God

It's me again

I believe ya

Be a wild one
Be a little dancer
Be the wind
Be the song on my lips
Be a snake in the marsh
Be a hand on the ivory keys
Be the one who chooses to bend her wings and take flight
Be the one in the sky
Be the kiss between lovers

MIHR, AGE 14

12

activism

Dear HIV, Why are you here?
Signed, Alan
Dear Alan, I am here to teach the world about human life.
Signed, HIV
—Alan, Age 16

What else can I say that will help you? What more do you need to hear? Have I said enough? I don't want to scare you too much. I want you to learn. About AIDS. About love. And about staying alive.

My friend Shaun once said,

"every miracle needs a little tending to."

It follows then that we must begin to see and nurture the miracles that we truly are, inviolate in our imperfections and flawless in our foibled ways. Remember the miracle and blessing of knowing the people that God has brought together. Continue to recognize the best within others so that we will learn to see the same within ourselves. Begin to collect pieces of goodness and compassion and offer them to each other. Pay attention to the lessons. Identify the blessings. And be willing to stay safe - willing to stay alive.

I talk to you because you carry the promise of life. When I leave you and the thousands of others that I speak to, there's hope in my heart that you'll stay alive forever. Sometimes I think that in twenty or thirty years from now, if I'm not alive anymore, you'll remember me, and talk about me, and you'll say that I've changed your lives in some way, that I helped to make it a little easier.

When I first found out about my HIV status, I didn't see beyond the age of thirty. On my thirtieth birthday, I set another goal. And I'll keep resetting it. But I'd rather focus on what I can do with my life today. And you are a part of it. Because it's no longer about what you want to be when you grow up. It's about who you are right now. What you can do in the meantime, with the rest of this day, as opposed to the rest of your lives?

I want the world to know you, and the good work that you are doing. I want your letters and poems and feelings to be revealed. I can see your fire. I can feel your fire. Yet when I hear that you and your peers are not looking out for yourselves and each other I get so angry.

AIDS has brought you into my life. Don't let AIDS take you away.

I've spoken to thousands and thousands of teenagers, and parents and teachers, yet there are still so many who are not listening, who just don't care, and who just don't think it's their problem. Part of me is frustrated and part of me knows that it's compassion they need because they're scared.

But they need something else. They need you.

I can't do all the work, I can't do it alone, and I can't do it forever. Help me. Do it with me. Make it your cause. For the time that we are here, let's get the message across to others that you can survive. You don't have to get infected, and you don't have to be too afraid.

Let's tell our teachers and our parents and our leaders, "Hey! I want to stay alive. So take responsibility and teach me everything I need to know. Everything!"

Just do the work. In a way this is so easy. All you have to do is open your hearts, get in touch with your feelings and just tell the truth. I see no other option at this point than to do anything else but love yourselves. I think it's all we ever have to do.

I'll make a promise to you if you make a promise to everybody else you speak to. Anyone and everyone. And make sure they promise you back:

I will stay alive if you will stay alive.

Promise them that you will take care of yourselves if they take care of themselves. If we could do that, we'd be working together. We'd be saying "Hey, I love you. I want you to stay around awhile." To the degree that you are brave in this world, you will surround yourself with others that are brave. And when you open up your heart, people will respond in kind. You can be the ones. That's what we call changing the world.

We are curing AIDS. Yes, this is a cure. We are here with each other. We are looking each other fully in the face. We're feeling, we're talking, were crying, we're hoping, we're praying, we're healing, we're curing.

We must learn to see AIDS not just as a disease but as a dark angel that breaks into our hearts in the middle of the night. We struggle as it wrests from us our faith in the future and our dreams of growing up. Yes we must fight. Yes we must do battle with it. And yes we will win. But we must not let it go unless we learn from it, unless it blesses us in some strange and even wonderful way. 🦋

MATT & HIS FRIENDS

Teenagers never stop talking. It's as if they need to be heard — if not by others, at least by themselves. To prove and proclaim, "Yeah, I get it, too! I understand." Like a yearning to be noticed and recognized; as if to say, "See me apart from the others. See how I love."

This evening, Matt came running over to me as I was eating my camp gruel in the dining hall. His voice was full of exclamation. He was noticeably out of breath and emotionally jolted.

"You'll never believe this! Never! I was outside, making a wish upon the first star I could see. And I promised myself I would never forget this moment, just like you told me to. But I couldn't find any stars. There were no stars anywhere. And as I was looking, all the time I was making my wish:

'I wish that they could find a cure for AIDS,'" Matt breathlessly announced. "When all of a sudden, out of nowhere, there was this huge flash of lightning and the entire sky lit up! And I swear to you, I knew that God was listening!"

Nearing the end of my travels, I harvested many gifts bestowed by charitable young-sters. It was a way to give back, I suppose, a little of what I had been giving them. I remember hearing my friend Don once say, "People want to believe in life. Their prayers for you are their 'thank you' for inspiring them."

A youngster named Sue approached me and gave me her necklace, saying, "You don't know me but the other day you told me you like this, so I want you to have it." Levi, thirteen, pulled me into his cabin to give me a "special something." "These are Vitamin C. They are good for your immune system. You should take these every day and you'll stay strong." After Ted heard that I lost my favorite denim shirt, one given to me by a friend who died of AIDS last year, he gave me one of his favorites to take its place. A group of older teens raised over $300 for me to donate, on their behalf, to the AIDS organization of my choice.

Friendship bracelets made of string and beads, gifts of cookies and kindness, poetry and prayers. And innocent admiration. All tendered from healing hands and generous hearts.

Abigail left me a note. "Life is running through you at full speed. Thank you for sharing that with me. I haven't felt this good or smiled this much in a while. Thank you for reminding me that there's so much to live. I hope you live a long and healthy life, and get to do all the things you want to."

Jonathan, who likes to call himself my "little brother," wrote, "I'm going to get serious for one brief moment. You really changed my life, and I don't know how to thank you. I know that if there is such a thing as heaven, you are on your way."

And an anonymous note simply said, "Thank you. You may have saved a life."

What I want is simple

I want to smile
Laugh, run, jump
Cry, hug, love
Kiss
Hold my best friends so tight that they moan

If I grow up
I want to be me

I want to fight
Hold hands, yell, scream, stomp
Sing, breathe, love

If I grow up
I want to be me

I want to swing, dance
Swim, punch, hit, eat and drink
Read, see, smell, touch
Hear and taste

If I grow up
I want to be me

I just want to live

ANNE, AGE 17

conclusion

Who says I am mortal? I want to live forever.
Will you try to stop me? I cannot be stopped.
I want to go against everything I've been taught. Is that so bad?

What if I wanted to fly?
If I were an eagle, would you tie my wings to the ground?

—Sara, Age 16

Often I think we carry secrets that we are born with, and though we sometimes twist and agonize at life's inconsistencies, the craving to reveal ourselves endures. Somehow we succeed. Certainly, every child and every teenager has a story to tell. Each knows a little something about the human existence. Each aches in his own way.

There's a sixteen year-old boy living outside of Miami having unprotected anal intercourse with a man more than twice his age. "I never had a father," he tells me. "He left when I was little and I'm looking for that missing presence in my life. I've thought about asking this guy to use a condom, but I always end up just letting him do what he wants. I need to have someone's arms around me, telling me he loves me." And then he adds, "I know what I'm doing is wrong, but I don't think I will stop."

There's a drama instructor at a camp in Pennsylvania who, as a child, was seduced by an older man in a dark alley. Because of his inner conflict and unresolved anger, he now believes he ambushed his feelings with years of "passionately violent sex."

There's a teenager in Washington DC, whose father sexually abused her in childhood. Now in college, she is uncomfortable to be naked in front of her boyfriend. "Every time he kisses me," she says, "I see my father's face."

And there's Annie from Australia, spending the summer as a counselor at a camp here in the United States. A few years ago, her nine year-old cousin was kidnaped, raped and drowned. Shari, sitting next to her, had three best friends who were killed in a car accident involving a drunk driver. Of their respective experiences, both say they simply shut down inside, blocked their emotions and acted out. "I just got drunk every night for weeks," Shari said.

Carly, from New Jersey, has Lupus. She came up to me at the end of one of my lectures to inquire, "How do you get out of bed in the morning? I ask because some mornings I can't even tie my shoes."

Elise is a lesbian. She is 19, in love and ready to marry Karen back home. This summer, she is teaching arts and crafts in a camp in the southeast. Afraid to be "found out", she has few friends and is cautious not to betray her recently claimed pride. "You know what's worse than coming out of the closet?" she asks, interrupting me to answer her own question. "Going back in."

Rebecca is sixteen years-old and from California. She raised her hand during one of my lectures. "I have this eye disease," she exclaimed aloud, through her tears, for the very first time in public. "And it means that one day I may not be able to see anymore. So, I've decided to see everything there is to see, before I can't see.

Melanie is a seventeen year-old who had an abortion last year. She and her boyfriend, both virgins, were having sex for the first time when she got pregnant. Sweet sixteen, she was worried that having an abortion might make her more susceptible to HIV infection. "No one understands me," she explains, "especially my parents."

Brian is a teenage hemophiliac with AIDS. "Do you know any teenagers who could be my friend?" he asks one night while sharing his root beer and apple pie with me. "I had all these friends in high school because they didn't know about my disease. But now I'm so sick and I'm afraid to tell them." He looks across the table at me and says, "You know...I just don't know if it's worth staying alive anymore."

Aubree, from Virginia, was afraid she might have infected her sex partners with HIV. She tells me that one night, in the middle of waiting three grueling weeks for her HIV test results, she was watching a television movie about a young woman dying from AIDS. Her father walked into the room and said, "Why are you wasting your time with that show? You know they only put it on to evoke sympathy." Fighting back her tears, she says to me, "It killed me. My father didn't know I was afraid that movie was gonna be about my life - that those very issues were right here in his home."

Tommy "froze inside for days" after he visited his ex-girlfriend in the hospital before she died of AIDS. Jamie's older sister's best friend, after testing positive for HIV, tried to kill himself by repeatedly stabbing his arm with a lead pencil. Joanna had a miscarriage after she was impregnated by a man who raped her. Hanah is sewing a memorial quilt panel for her father who died of AIDS. Traci is afraid to trust anyone. Timothy has lost his faith in God. And Kathy is lonely.

Why do teenagers put themselves at risk for HIV infection? Most say of themselves, "It can't happen to me." Others don't want to think of the consequences or accept the responsibilities of sex. Some teenagers don't want to surrender their passion in the heat of the moment while others have low self-esteem and are not able to speak up for themselves. For some, safer sex is awkward and awkwardness can lead to vulnerability and intimacy, and intimacy can be scary. Many teenagers foolishly still think AIDS is a homosexual disease and that "guys can't get it from girls." Some teens choose to be rebellious and say, "Who cares, we're all gonna die anyway?" and others are simply too drunk to resist the easy urge. Many think, "it's not cool to wear a condom." Some are more concerned with not getting pregnant. There are youngsters that are still not properly educated or are naive while others go against everything they are taught. And so on and so on.

But I believe there is yet another reason. Could it be that these youngsters sense the true delicateness of invincibility? Have they been deceived in their belief in a life of invulnerability? Ironically, they are taught that these are the "best years of their lives," while grief or pain invariably, in one form or another, asserts itself. In this generation of AIDS, we must begin to recognize that teenagers are being prematurely greeted by, and are unprepared for, life's faithful aches.

Teens are the overlooked heroes — the sometimes inarticulate people in pain who swallow their sorrow, fear and confusion with self-neglect in the forms of drugs, alcohol and unsafe sex. AIDS in their community exists as a manifestation of an even greater disease: growing up in a society that fosters a lack of survival skills, like high self-esteem, self-respect, self-discipline and most especially, self-love. I contend that once they are given the room to acknowledge their difficult journey and the praise they deserve for their efforts, there is a chance they will recognize their value and self-worth and fully participate in protecting their futures. As one teen put it, "I get it. I value my life. And if I hurt myself, then I hurt all the people around me who love me." And in the words of another, "We need to feel the value of our own lives. If we don't acknowledge that, giving it all up to ignorance or weakness becomes easy." And still another, "We must remember that it's not our bodies that are indestructible, but our spirits."

There is a modern Hebrew song by David Broza that goes, "y'hiyeh tov, y'hiyeh tov cain, lifamim ani nishbar." Translated to English, it means, "It will be fine, it will be fine, yes. Even though at times I am broken." As I listen to the stories of these brave youngsters, I attempt to help them find room inside to be at peace with being broken.

I remember a flower that my friend Deborah once put in front of me. We studied it with reverence for its silence, its dignity and its perfection. We noticed how it never complained or wondered if it was anything less than beautiful. And suddenly, a single petal fell to the table. "See," said Deborah, "even the flower is falling apart." To which I replied, "And it is no less beautiful, no less perfect."

And I remember a piece of a prayer I once read that went something like, "Dear God, please cherish our fragmented hearts."

As I look upon these faces of summer, I wonder how I can teach these teenagers to cherish what feels like a heart fragmented. Perhaps true healing comes not from asking God to cover our blemishes or to put us back together again, but from honoring and respecting some of the inner torment, bearing witness to life's lessons. I endeavor to teach these teens how to recognize the sweetness in the fragility of their lives and how to salute each other for continuing to seek gladness, in spite of life's demanding circumstances.

They are champions, these teenagers — young soldiers of survival in a common battle, defending the innocence of simple joys. They get out of bed each morning with aspirations and promises renewed. They fight over seconds for dessert, dream of getting behind the wheel of a car for the very first time, and talk about their first kiss. Some still love to be sung to sleep, while others wait for full moons. With hearts full of bounty, they illuminate the simple but deep joy of feeling alive, as if to say, "Thanks, God. I get it. That full moon is shining just for me."

While I sang the lullaby to the Shoafim girls that July night, fourteen year-old Andrea, in a darkened corner furtively lit by a flashlight, was writing an elegy under the covers of her bottom bunk-bed.

Is summer laughter sweeter

When autumn's cold touch threatens to obscure

The warm song of youth?

Does knowledge that death exists

Make life all the more joyful

To one whose mornings might end too soon?

Does approaching twilight

Add the poignant joy-sadness

To the last day of summer?

I learn from you not how to die

But how to live

During my travels this summer, I met an elderly woman who lived through the Holocaust of Nazi Germany. She was relating her story of survival to a group of weary campers in the sweltering Pennsylvania heat. She was demonstrating the strength, resilience and indestructibility of the human spirit.

She told the youngsters that she never cried in those days. "Though there was always time to be afraid," she said, "there was no time for tears. I was too hungry and too busy trying to survive."

"Let me tell you something," she continued. "You can live three weeks without food, three days without water. But without hope, you will not live even three minutes."

She expressed her faith that this generation will make the difference. I believe this as well. These youthful aspirers, nourished by hope, share an infatuation with life. Certainly passion — though at times temporarily muted, and at others, forthright and loud — is thriving inside each of them.

———

This has been a summer of miracles. As August's evening wind brushes branches against the backdrop of a pastel-colored sky, I think back upon the lectures I've given, the poems I've gathered, and the people I've met.

As I've traveled from camp to camp, all the things I have needed and known have been within reach: the dining room up the hill, the rec hall down the road, the bunks beyond the woods. And thousands of teenagers, laughing and screaming. Surviving. Thriving. Somehow, the "outside world" seems heavier. Indeed, there is a lightness that comes from loving.

It is difficult saying goodbye to a season of youngsters who carry fledgling promises that they'll never forget the goodness of these days. I listen to stories and songs on a soft summer night. I am on a lake in the rain, dancing in a rowboat with the "tough boys of Bunk 15" as they tell me how much I make them cry and feel and want to sing. A teenager, named Jason, slips me a note which says, "I want you to know you were there for me when I was too afraid to see help – now I'll always be there for you."

And I want to capture all of it in my cerebral diary and share it with the world.

One teen, walking past me, tearfully exclaims to her best friend, "I just want to stay with you for as long as I can."

In the sage words of another, "The living, breathing flesh holds no bounds for the infinite creativity which lies within."

And finally, Debbie from Miami, with adolescent sagacity keeps reminding me, "It's all good. It's all good."

So I race up hills with them. I collect their poems and prayers under promising skies. And I share nocturnal giggles as we affirm our will to survive. We are "the aspirers," proclaiming together the majesty of life, as we race under the moon. ❧